Applying MBA Knowledge and Skills to Healthcare

Applying MBA Knowledge and Skills to Healthcare

Reza Nassab
Plastic Surgery Registrar
Whiston Hospital, Liverpool

Vaikunthan Rajaratnam
Consultant Hand Surgeon
The Royal Orthopaedic Hospital, Birmingham

and

Michael Loh
Executive Consultant
IBM Global Services, Singapore

Foreword by
B Sonny Bal
Associate Professor of Orthopaedic Surgery
University of Missouri School of Medicine, Missouri

Radcliffe Publishing
London • New York

Radcliffe Publishing Ltd
33–41 Dallington Street
London
EC1V 0BB
United Kingdom

www.radcliffepublishing.com

Electronic catalogue and worldwide online ordering facility.

British Library Cataloguing in Publication Data

A catalogue record for this book is available from the British Library.

ISBN-13: 978 184619 375 0

Typeset by Phoenix Photosetting, Chatham, Kent
Printed and bound by Cadmus Communications, USA

Contents

Foreword   xi

About the authors   xiii

List of abbreviations   xv

Introduction   **1**
So what is management?   1
How is management applicable to clinical practice?   1
The anatomy of management   2

Module 1: Accounting and finance   **5**
Accounting   5
Finance   5
Company law requirements for financial accounts   6
The accounting formula   6
    Assets   7
    Equity   7
    Liabilities   7
Balance sheet   8
Profit and loss account   9
Cash flow statement   10
Ratio analysis   11
Summary   12
References   12
Useful websites   12

Module 2: Operations management   **13**
Managing all the activities required to create and deliver your goods
    or services   13
Substantial measurement and analysis of processes   14
    Speed   14
    Dependability   14
    Flexibility   15
    Cost   15

    Quality   15
Employment of methods to improve performance   18
    Six Sigma   18
    Lean   20
    Lean Six Sigma   21
    Process re-engineering   22
Summary   24
Exercises   24
Sample answer for process re-engineering   25
References   26
Case studies   26
Further reading   27
Useful websites   27

Module 3: Marketing in healthcare   **28**
Marketing and healthcare   28
Marketing process   29
Analysis of marketing opportunities   29
Selecting target markets   31
Developing the marketing mix   32
Product   32
    Product life cycle   32
Price   34
Place   34
Promotion   35
People   36
Managing the marketing effort   36
Summary   37
Exercises   37
Sample answer for a marketing plan   38
References   40
Further reading   41
Useful websites   41

Module 4: Strategic management for clinicians   **42**
Strategy   42
Objective setting   42
Analysis   43
SWOT analysis   43
Porter's five forces   43
    Threat of entry   45
    Threat of substitutes   45
    Power of suppliers   45
    Power of buyers   46
    Competitive rivalry   46

PESTEL   47
Plan   47
    Porter's strategies   47
    Ansoff product-growth matrix   49
Implementation   50
Evaluation and control   50
Summary   50
Exercises   51
References   51
Further reading   51

Module 5: Information technology (IT)   **53**
Patient care   53
Imaging   55
Personal development   56
Research and information   56
Online education   57
Scheduling   57
Social networking   57
    Blogs   58
    Facebook   58
    Twitter   58
Organisational   59
Summary   59
Exercises   59
References   60
Further reading   60
Useful websites   60

Module 6: Human resource management   **61**
Strategic human resource management   61
Requirements   61
Workforce planning   62
Recruitment   63
    Job design   63
    Job description   63
    Recruitment process   64
Reward management   64
Retention   64
Summary   67
Exercises   68
References   68
Case studies   68
Further reading   68
Useful websites   68

Module 7: The clinical team   **69**
Anatomy of a team   70
   Independent teams (surgeons operating)   70
   Interdependent teams (the surgical team)   70
The physiology of the clinical team   70
   Forming stage   70
   Storming stage   71
   Norming state   71
   Performing stage   71
   Adjourning stage   72
Team roles   72
Building effective teams   73
Team effectiveness model   73
Team dynamics   73
Delegation   74
Conflict   75
   Types of conflict   75
   Conflict process   75
Why the clinical team?   78
Working examples of a clinical team   79
Summary   79
Exercises   79
References   80
Further reading   80
Useful websites   80

Module 8: Clinical leaders   **81**
Study of leadership   81
   Trait approach   81
   Behaviour approach   82
   Power-influence approach   83
   Situational approach   83
   Integrative approach   83
Transactional and transformational leadership   83
Becoming a transformational leader   85
Mentoring and coaching   86
   Mentoring   86
   Coaching   88
Summary   89
Exercises   89
References   89
Case studies   90
Further reading   90
Useful websites   90

Module 9: Managing clinicians' performance 91
Defining performance 91
What do we measure? 91
Patient pathway 92
Key performance indicators for clinicians 93
What matters most? 94
Why manage performance? 94
Who drives performance? 94
    Doctor 94
    Patients 95
    Regulatory bodies 96
    Financiers of healthcare 96
    Management 97
How to manage doctors' performance 97
Summary 99
Exercises 100
References 100
Case example 101
Useful websites 101

Module 10: The learning and teaching clinician 102
Learning 102
    Experiential learning model 102
Types of learner 103
Learning event planning 105
    Needs assessment 105
    Objectives 107
    Target audience 107
    Approach 107
    Delivery 109
    Evaluation 110
Summary 110
Exercises 111
Sample answer for training event 112
References 114
Further reading 114
Useful websites 114

Module 11: Coping with change in the clinical environment 115
Change management 115
    People 115
    Organisational culture 117
    Processes 118
Why does change fail? 119
Leading a successful change initiative 119

Summary   121
Exercises   122
References   122
Further reading   122
Useful websites   122

Module 12: Innovation in medicine   **123**
The innovative healthcare organisation   124
The innovative management   125
The innovative doctor   125
Exercises   127
References   127
Further reading   127
Useful websites   127

Glossary   128

Index   131

Foreword

Beyond medical knowledge, clinicians increasingly need a strong grasp of the fundamental principles of business management, organisational structure, finance and related subjects that are traditionally taught during a graduate business education, and seldom (if ever) addressed during medical training. Like other disciplines, medical care has changed drastically in the last 25 years, and the idea of gaining business acumen while running a medical practice is no longer practical.

During the past several years, an increasing number of clinicians have found it worthwhile to supplement their medical training with a formal exposure to business school. However, the costs and time commitments related to a business education, once a physician is already in practice or even before that time, are formidable. A number of authors have sought to write about the business principles that clinicians should be familiar with; most such attempts reflect a rather dry and formalistic approach to enlightening clinicians about business and its related principles.

Applying MBA Knowledge and Skills to Healthcare has taken a welcome approach in that rather than preach to physicians about business school principles, the authors have invested the time to present information in a practical, actionable format. As the title suggests, this is a practical primer on applications of MBA principles to clinical practice. Busy clinicians, academic surgeons, administrative physicians and other healthcare professionals will find this book to be an invaluable resource in understanding the core principles of business management, and in learning how to apply them; the target audience is indeed very broad.

A particular strength of the book is the lucid, tight organisation of complex subjects into modules; much like a business education might be structured. In 12 well-written modules, the authors have managed to cover the entire gamut of a business education; from basic finance and accounting principles, to more esoteric subjects such as strategic management methods, and leadership theories. It is rare to find a book that is written with brevity, focus, clarity and precision; while the topics are serious, the reading is never weary or burdensome. For busy clinicians, the value proposition is enormous in terms of the knowledge gained, versus the amount of reading required to capture what the authors have so capably managed to distil between the covers.

Medical students and physicians-in-training would be one natural audience for this book since it imparts necessary skills and knowledge that are best gained during the formative years in medicine. Experienced clinicians, and even those with a formal MBA business education, such as me, will find this book to be a succinct, welcome refresher on the fundamentals of business principles. The authors have done a remarkable task in capturing the latest concepts and thinking in the business management arena, while adding useful and eclectic topics such as *Innovation in medicine* (Module 12), and *Managing the clinician's performance* (Module 9). The authors have managed to capture the essence of an entire MBA education, and customise it for healthcare professionals.

True to the style of a business education, each module is structured with helpful exercises at the end, encouraging reader participation, and creating intellectual challenges and stimulation. Hopefully, future versions of this text will maintain the attractive style of writing, the engaging prose and the economy of words that make this a delight, and a strong recommendation to healthcare professionals worldwide. This text will be especially welcome where the medical profession faces fast-paced, unprecedented change. Enlightened by this book, the reader will be able to spot opportunity in that change.

B Sonny Bal, MD, JD, MBA
Associate Professor
Department of Orthopaedic Surgery
University of Missouri
Columbia, MO
February 2011

About the authors

Reza Nassab
MBChB, MBA, MRCSEd, MRCSEng
Plastic Surgery Registrar, Mersey Deanery

Mr Nassab graduated from the University of Birmingham Medical School in 2000 and has subsequently worked in Nottingham, Birmingham and London. He completed his basic surgical training and became a member of the Royal College of Surgeons of England and Edinburgh. He is currently a trainee plastic surgeon in the Mersey region. During his clinical work, he undertook a MBA degree at Aston University, from which he graduated in March 2008. His dissertation for this degree explored leadership and personality traits amongst plastic surgeons. Mr Nassab has published many peer-reviewed articles in a number of well-respected international journals. He has also presented at many national and international meetings.

Vaikunthan Rajaratnam
MBBS (Mal), AM (Mal), FRCS (Ed), FRCS (Glasg), FICS (USA), MBA (USA), Dip Hand Surgery (Eur), PG CertMedEd (Dundee), FHEA (UK)
Consultant Hand Surgeon, The Royal Orthopaedic Hospital, Birmingham

Mr Rajaratnam, Consultant Hand Surgeon working in the National Health Service in the United Kingdom, has more than 25 years' experience in teaching and training doctors and medical undergraduates. He is an accredited hand surgeon and medical educator with numerous research presentation and publications in hand surgery, surgical education and management in medicine. He is a Fellow of the Higher Education Academy UK and has a medical education qualification from Dundee with an MBA. He is the prime mover for two Masters programmes in hand therapy and professional administration, having developed the curriculum and e-learning course management systems. He has also worked as a management consultant to the insurance industry in developing systems for medical fraud prevention.

Michael Loh
Executive Consultant, Integrated Technology Delivery, Geo Service Delivery, IBM Global Services, ASEAN

Dr Loh is an acknowledged authority on the psychology of change and a recognised expert on organisation development. He is a diplomate of the American Association of Psychotherapists, a life member of the National Psychiatric Association, USA, and member of L'Association Internationale de Psychologie Appliquee, as well as a Professional Member of the American Counselling Association. He has been elected to the President's Council of the American Institute of Management. Dr Loh is also a Certified Management Consultant. In addition, he has been awarded the designation Certified Professional Consultant to Management by the National Bureau of Certified Consultants, USA. Dr Loh has lectured on MBA programs for University of South Australia, University of Western Sydney, University of Hull (UK), Burapha University (Thailand), and University of Luton (UK). Dr Loh has also recently published his fifth book.

List of abbreviations

AMA	American Medical Association
CDC	Centre for Diseases Control and Prevention
CIPD	Chartered Institute of Personnel and Development
CIRO	Context, Inputs, Reactions, Outcomes
CME	Continuing medical education
CPD	Continuing professional development
DMAIC	Define, Measure, Analyse, Improve, Control
EHCR	Electronic healthcare record
EMR	Electronic medical record
GMC	General Medical Council
GP	General practitioner (family physician)
IT	Information technology
KPI	Key performance indicator
KSA	Knowledge, Skills and Ability
NHS	National Health Service
PACS	Picture archiving and communications system
PAS	Patient administration system
PBL	Problem based learning
PCPI	Physician Consortium for Performance Improvement
PESTEL	Political, Economic, Social, Technological, Environmental, Legal
SCU	Strategic clinical unit
SHRM	Strategic human resource management
SMART	Specific, Measurable, Agreed, Realistic, Time Based
SWOT	Strengths, Weaknesses, Opportunities, Threats
VLE	Virtual learning environment

Dedicated to my parents Javad and Parvin

For providing me with the opportunity to become who I am today

RN

*To all those who have known me and tolerated my constant ramblings.
Hopefully I have had an iota of positive impact and will likewise impact
others.*

Be enlightened that you may enlighten

VR

*To my wife, Dr Tan Gek Inn, whose continuous support continues to fuel the
pursuit of my dreams*

ML

Introduction

Medicine is an ever-evolving profession that impacts on one's life beyond expectations. During medical training we are taught skills that will enable us to proceed through our desired career paths. Medical courses have evolved with time and the emphasis has been removed from basic sciences and placed more on the social sciences and communication. In this ever-changing world of medicine we see medical advances that have given us unrivalled insights into disease processes, diagnostics and their management. As we progress throughout our life long journey into the world of medicine, we also begin to see the increasing importance of management in medicine. Many of us see management as restrictive to our progress, proving to be an obstacle in our journey. Management must not, however, be viewed upon in this way. If you pick up any newspaper, you will see stories of businesses and their leaders who have captured the world with their products and services. Their successes and failures provide us with valuable knowledge and skills that may be applied to our way of life. Management and business does not purely revolve around the financial markets, stock exchanges and banking organisations. Management principles are readily applicable to many situations faced by medical professionals. An insight into management also gives practitioners opportunities to develop skills and enhance the provision of care. The emergence of dual medical and management degrees reinforces the significant impact of management in the future of medicine.

So what is management?

Management may be defined as:

> *The organisational process that involves managing resources, inclusive of human and financial assets, needed to achieve the objectives of the organisation, and monitoring the outcomes. Management also includes recording and storing facts and information for strategic use. Managerial tasks are not limited to managers or supervisors but every member of the organisation.*

How is management applicable to clinical practice?

For medical practitioners management is about effective utilisation of time and effort in achieving the collective goals of their practice. The process requires definition of our goals and achievement of these in a timely manner. Execution of this needs a team approach effectively directed by a leader. Achievement of goals and targets is monitored and adjustments made to improve performance. This is analogous to the clinical model of gathering clinical information, performing investigations and formulating a diagnosis and treatment plan with your clinical team. The treatment is then monitored to ensure the desired agreed outcomes are achieved effectively and efficiently.

The anatomy of management

The modern day practice of management comprises a number of core disciplines, which include the following.

1 Accounting and finance.
2 Operations.
3 Marketing.
4 Strategy.
5 Information technology (IT).
6 Human resources.
7 Change and innovation.

This book is structured into modules covering these core management disciplines. Each module will explore the discipline and demonstrate how it can be applied to a clinical setting. The reader can explore each module independently of the others, but you will soon see how the modules become interrelated.

Accounting and finance

Clinicians must have a basic understanding of accounting and finance. Whether it is private or public sector, money is a key driver in the provision of healthcare. Using accounting and financial principles, we can formulate records highlighting our resources, expenses and incomes. Based on this information, we can use techniques, such as ratio analysis, to assess performance. Therefore, we can summarise thus.

➤ What resources do we have?
➤ How should we allocate resources?
➤ Are the resources being used efficiently?

Operations

Operations management explores how an organisation is run on a daily basis and the processes involved. When providing any service or product, there are many stages in its production, distribution and delivery. Operations management looks closely at all these stages and allows us to answer the following questions.

➤ What are the stages of providing a service or product?
➤ How can we measure and analyse the performance of each stage?
➤ What steps can we employ to improve our performance?
➤ How can we maintain and improve performance and quality?

Many of you will have already undertaken an operations management project without realising it. The most common example in medicine is the clinical audit cycle.

Within the cycle, we identify a service that we are providing and measure current performance. We compare this with the acceptable or gold standards. Methods to improve the service and achieve these standards are then introduced. Finally, measurement of performance is undertaken to analyse if we have achieved the desired performance.

Marketing

Many will consider marketing to be about advertising and selling a product. Although this is partly true, there is a lot more to marketing. Marketing is the process of ensuring products and services are produced and delivered to the appropriate recipients to satisfy their needs. Marketing principles are applicable to all sectors of healthcare, such as private, public or research. In the public sector, health promotion campaigns are an excellent example of marketing in action. When considering any marketing solution, we must answer the following questions.

➤ What are the gaps or opportunities in the market?
➤ Who is the target of our product or service?
➤ What are their specific needs?
➤ How can we address their needs?
➤ How can we differentiate our product or service?
➤ How can we maintain our position in the market?

Strategy

A strategy is a plan of action designed to achieve a particular goal or outcome. This can be anything from developing a vision for an organisation as a whole to the launch of a new product or service. A strategic plan addresses the following questions.

➤ Where are we?
➤ Where do we want to be?
➤ How and when do we get there?
➤ Why do we want to be there?
➤ What is involved in getting there?
➤ What are the obstacles we may encounter?
➤ How are we going to assess if we made it?

Reading this list of questions, one can see it is readily applicable to any situation that we may come across. The module will cover some specific tools and techniques frequently employed by strategists to answer these questions.

Information technology

Information technology has now become an integral part of any organisation, especially in healthcare. This ensures that all systems and processes in an organisation work to provide access to information and data when it is required. This can include patient care, imaging, research, and administrative information. In this module, we shall look at what resources are currently available to enable efficient and effective use of information technology in an organisation.

Human resources

Arguably the most important component of any healthcare organisation is the providers of the service. Human resources encompasses many aspects of dealing with employees including the following.

➤ Requirement, recruitment and retention of employees.
➤ Teamwork.
➤ Leadership.
➤ Measuring performance.
➤ Learning, training and development.

Change and innovation

Innovation and change may often be considered to coexist. Innovation has driven medical science and our ability to treat disease. Promoting innovation improves patient care. Change must happen to take on board innovative ideas. In these modules we shall explore factors that help make change within organisations and individuals more acceptable. We shall also discuss ways of encouraging innovative thinking.

Accounting and finance

Finance may be considered as the heart of any organisation, which requires cash flow to circulate throughout it to provide other parts with resources to maintain their vitality. Understanding financial basics is crucial for any managerial role within an organisation. We shall explore basic terms and techniques used in finance and illustrate these with examples. So let's start with the definitions, as there is often confusion between accounting and finance.

Accounting is basically the system of making records, verifications and reporting of the value of assets, liabilities, expenses and income in the account books. The transactions are posted chronologically to record changes in value of assets and liabilities. It is the process of collecting and recording data about the use of funds within an organisation. The clinical analogy is the collection of blood and biopsy to make diagnoses and how they are recorded in the clinical notes.

Accounting

There are two types accounting for an organisation.

➤ **Financial accounting** – focuses on information for people outside the firm. These may include creditors and outside investors, who are not part of the day-to-day management of the company. Government agencies and the general public are external users that may be interested in accounting information.
➤ **Management accounting** – focuses on information for internal decision makers, such hospital administrators.

Finance

Finance refers to the time, money and risk associated with a specific business. Finance differs because it works on the accounting information to predict future trends or to make decisions about the future. This is analogous to clinical medicine, where, through your history, examination and investigations, you make a clinical decision based on calculated risk to treat your patient. Finance is concerned with the raising of funds to meet the various cash flow needs of the organisation. Finance functions start from gathering the cash flow information from the accounting records and preparing projections of cash flow. Finance activities are concerned with preparing budgets, undertaking comparisons and finding variances. Finance activities therefore will encompass both the accounting and operations aspects of an organisation.

Company law requirements for financial accounts

Every UK Company registered under the Companies Act is required to prepare a set of accounts that give a true and fair view of its profit or loss for the year and of its state of affairs at the year-end.

Annual accounts for Companies Act purposes generally include the following.

➤ **Directors' report** – Description by the directors of the performance of the business during the accounting period + various additional disclosures, particularly in relation to directors' shareholdings, remuneration, etc.
➤ **Balance sheet** – Statement of assets and liabilities at the end of the accounting period (a 'snapshot') of the business.
➤ **Profit and loss account** – Describing the trading performance of the business over the accounting period.
➤ **Statement of total recognised gains and losses.**
➤ **Cash flow statement** – Describing the cash inflows and outflows during the accounting period.
➤ **Audit report.**
➤ **Notes to the accounts** – Additional details that have to be disclosed to comply with Accounting Standards and the Companies Act.

In England, the accounts of an NHS foundation trust must comply with International Financial Reporting Standards (IFRS) as adopted by the European Union. All private healthcare organisations have to comply by the company law requirements.

In the United States, companies can become limited liability companies, incorporated or corporations. The exact terminology used varies depending on the requirements and from state to state. The corporate business law also varies between different states. Limited liability companies tend to have less legal requirements and formalities than corporations.

The three main financial statements outlined in the above legal requirements are therefore:

➤ balance sheet
➤ profit and loss account
➤ cash flow statement.

We shall look at these individually and examine their components and composition. In order to illustrate these principles, we shall present a case study of a fictional company.

The accounting formula

The basis of accounting revolves around the formula shown in Figure 1.1.

This equation has three components, which are as follows.

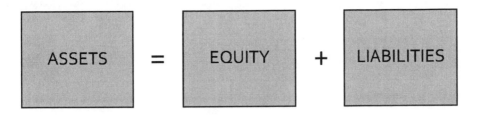

Figure 1.1: The accounting formula

Assets

These are the rights and things that a company owns. They can be classified as either current or fixed assets. This is determined by the liquidity of the assets. Liquidity can be described as the ability to settle costs with cash or assets that can be promptly converted to cash. In this case, current assets are things that can be converted into cash within a year. Current assets include stock, cash and trade debtors (money owed to you). Fixed assets are intended for long-term or continuing use to allow the organisation to conduct its business. Fixed assets may be classified into tangible and intangible. Tangible fixed assets include land, property, machinery and vehicles. With time the value of these fixed assets will reduce – this is called depreciation. For instance, a hospital purchases a MRI scanner but the life span of this machine is limited. Over the life span of the scanner its value reduces. There are differing techniques to account for depreciation and seeking professional advice is recommended. Intangible fixed assets are things such as goodwill, patents, copyrights and brands an organisation may possess.

Equity

In order to acquire assets, an organisation needs to obtain cash from differing sources. Equity or capital is the cash invested into the company by its owners or shareholders.

Liabilities

Further cash is acquired from other sources such as bank loans. These are borrowings the company owes, which are referred to as liabilities. These can again be classified into current and long-term liabilities. The differentiation between the two depends on the duration over which the liability is owed. Short-term liabilities may include money owed to suppliers, short-term loans or taxes due. Therefore, if a company owes something within a year this is a current liability and beyond a year it becomes a long-term liability. Examples of long-term liabilities include bank loans and finance agreements due to be repaid after one year.

Now the components of the accounting formula have been defined, we can see how they make up the balance sheet.

Case study

HealMe Limited was established almost a year ago and produces a medicinal preparation that when applied to a wound helps the healing process. The company was set up by a small group of friends who had invested a significant amount of their own money. They needed additional funding and approached their bank for a loan, which was granted. Using their initial investment they purchased a factory and machinery to produce their product.

Balance sheet

The balance sheet is a statement of an organisation's assets, equity and liabilities at a particular date, which is usually the last date of the accounting period. This provides an overview of how the organisation is being funded and how the funds are being utilised (*see* Figure 1.2).

The balance sheet for HealMe Limited illustrates the main three components, which are assets, liabilities and equity. In this example, the fixed assets (such as property and machinery) are valued at £300 000. Current assets are also available

BALANCE SHEET OF HEALME LIMITED

		£ (THOUSAND)
FIXED ASSETS		300
CURRENT ASSETS		
STOCK	40	
DEBTORS	30	
CASH	20	
TOTAL	90	
CURRENT LIABILITIES	(50)	40
NET ASSETS		340
SHARE EQUITY		200
RETAINED PROFIT		140
EQUITY EMPLOYED		340

Figure 1.2: Balance sheet

totalling £90 000. The company has some current liabilities, which are deducted resulting in a net asset of £340 000. Equity comes from the investment by shares and also some retained profit. The value of this equity should, according to our equation, be equal to assets less liabilities. This statement therefore balances.

Profit and loss account

This statement summarises the organisation's trading transactions, which comprise income, sales and expenses. This statement is also based on an equation (*see* Figure 1.3). Profit should be one of the primary drivers for any organisation. The profit and loss account looks at transactions over a period of time, unlike the balance sheet that only provides a snapshot at a particular time.

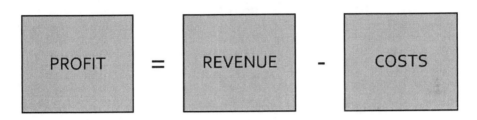

Figure 1.3: The profit formula

Using the equation, we can see profit may be increased either by increasing revenue or by decreasing costs. Revenue is generated from turnover or sales. Costs can be incurred in many ways and it is often useful to classify costs. Costs can therefore be of the following kind.

➤ **Fixed costs** – These are costs incurred over a period irrespective of the level of output or resources used. For example, the cost of owning or renting a property, insurance and professional memberships.
➤ **Variable costs** – Variable costs, as the name implies, vary depending on the level of activity. Hence, electricity bills or raw material costs may be significantly higher during periods of high production.
➤ **Opportunity costs** – These are opportunities that were not pursued in favour of the chosen product or service. To illustrate this concept, we use an example of a hospital that decides to invest in building a new ward but had the opportunity to buy a new scanner. The opportunity cost would be the revenue generated from the scanner and avoiding having to outsource scans to another hospital.
➤ **Sunk costs** – Sunk costs are costs that have been incurred that cannot be recovered. A simple example may be purchasing a ticket and missing the train.

Using the profit and loss statement for HealMe Limited (*see* Figure 1.4), we can look at its structure, which is closely related to our profit equation. In this statement, the company had a turnover of £500 000. We must then consider the costs encountered and so firstly we have the cost of goods sold. This is the cost directly incurred in

PROFIT AND LOSS STATEMENT OF HEALME LIMITED

FOR PERIOD APRIL 2009 TO APRIL 2010

	£ (THOUSAND)
TURNOVER (SALES)	500
LESS COST OF GOODS SOLD	(200)
GROSS PROFIT	300
LESS OTHER COSTS	(100)
OPERATING PROFIT	200
TAX	(40)
PROFIT AFTER TAX	160
DIVIDENDS	20
RETAINED PROFIT	140
	160

Figure 1.4: Profit and loss statement

the production of the good to be sold. Direct costs include materials and labour. Deduction of this cost gives us the gross profit. We have other indirect costs, such as marketing and research, which are then deducted to give the operating profit. We must also deduct tax, which then gives us the net profit.

Profit can then be either retained for future investment or paid back to shareholders in the form of dividends.

Cash flow statement

The cash flow statement records all inflows and outflows of cash over a period (*see* Figure 1.5). Within the cash flow statement, transactions are included only when the cash has be paid or received, as opposed to the profit and loss statement that includes all transactions. This varies from the profit and loss statement, which takes into account factors such as depreciation. Cash flow statements provide a more accurate reflection of transactions.

The cash flow statement for our company (*see* Figure 1.5) reveals a more detailed breakdown of incomes and expenses. This allows calculation of the net cash flow. This statement is useful for assessing the solvency or liquidity of a company. These are measures of whether a company is capable of meeting its long- and short-term obligations, respectively. The statement also allows us to identify trends cash flows and therefore making adjustments according to these trends.

CASH FLOW STATEMENT OF HEALME LIMITED

FOR PERIOD APRIL 2009 TO JUNE 2009

£ (THOUSAND)

	APRIL	MAY	JUNE
INCOME			
CASH SALES	300	200	400
DEBTOR PAYMENTS	30	30	30
TOTAL INCOME	270	230	430
EXPENSES			
MATERIALS	200	300	100
WAGES	30	30	30
BILLS	20	20	20
TOTAL EXPENSES	250	350	150
NET CASH FLOW	20	-120	280
OPENING BALANCE	200	220	100
NET CASH FLOW	20	-120	280
CLOSING BALANCE	220	100	380

Figure 1.5: Cash flow statement

Ratio analysis

Ratio analysis provides a useful method of using figures from the financial statements to calculate an organisation's performance. There are four main methods of ratio analysis.

➤ **Liquidity ratios** – Provide an indication of the capability of an organisation to meet its short-term obligations. For example, the acid-ratio is calculated by dividing current assets (excluding stock) by current liabilities. A ratio of one shows high liquidity and hence good financial health.

➤ **Solvency ratios** – Allow a measure of an organisation to meet its long-term obligations. The gearing ratio is the contribution of owner's equity to long-term liabilities. It is calculated by dividing all long-term liabilities by shareholder equity. The higher the level of borrowing (or gearing), the more vulnerable the company is to increasing interest rates.

➤ **Efficiency ratios** – Allow an insight into how efficiently resources are invested into fixed assets and working capital. An example includes stock turnover (average cost of sales divided by average value of stock), which indicates how long one should hold one's stock before selling.

➤ **Profitability ratios** – Provide an assessment of whether a business is making a profit. The gross profit margin is the gross profit divided by the revenue. Other profitability ratios include return on capital employed.

Summary

Accounting and finance are the heart of any organisation. We have seen how organisations are legally required to produce statements of their financial activities. The three main statements include the balance sheet, cash flow statement and the profit and loss statement. Based on these statements, we can use accounting techniques to assess various aspects of an organisation such its efficiency and profitability. This module is intended to be an introduction of accounting and should form a good grounding for understanding the basics. Specialist advice should always be sought, as there are many complexities in accounting terminology and practices.

References

1   Chadwick L. *Essential Finance and Accounting for Managers*. Harlow: Pearson Education Ltd; 2002.
2   Mott G. *Accounting for Non-Accountants*. 7th ed. London: Kogan Page; 2008.

Useful websites

Business Link: www.businesslink.gov.uk
Tutor2u – Accounting and Finance: http://tutor2u.net/sub_accounting.asp

Operations management

When a medical professional is asked about operations, the image of a surgeon in the theatre undertaking a procedure on a patient will be the one that immediately comes to mind. This surgical procedure may be considered as an operations process. Operations management consists of the following.

➤ Managing all the activities required to create and deliver your goods or services.
➤ Substantial measurement and analysis of processes.
➤ Employment of methods to improve performance.

Managing all the activities required to create and deliver your goods or services

The basis of an operations process is transforming a set of 'inputs' into 'output' goods or services for the end user (*see* Figure 2.1).[1]

Figure 2.1 simplifies the overall process into three main components. The inputs, that can be divided broadly into two categories, which are the transformed resources and transforming resources. First, the transformed resources are all raw materials, information and clients that are involved in the operation process. Secondly, the transforming resources are the facilities and staff required for the transformation process. The next stage is the transformation process, which involves processing of all inputs to produce the goods or service, also known as the output. At each stage, a significant number of other processes are taking place that all require monitoring and analysis to ensure efficient and effective production of outputs.

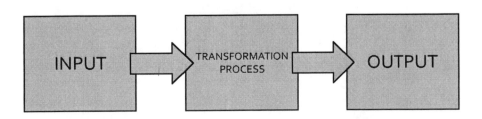

Figure 2.1: The typical operations process

As clinicians, we are undertaking operations management on a daily basis. A patient (transformed resource) enters the practice or hospital and is treated by staff and facilities (transforming resources). The treatment results in a transformation process for the patient and a service is provided, whether it is prescription of medication, investigation or invasive intervention (output). During each of the stages, we can monitor the provision of treatment, assess outcomes and identify any need for improvements.

Substantial measurement and analysis of processes

In order to measure and analyse processes we need defined objectives. There are five main performance objectives (*see* Figure 2.2).[1]

Speed

Speed is determined by the period of time from customer request to delivery of product and service. In medicine, this can be interpreted as the time taken from referral to treat a patient.

Dependability

Dependability means provision or delivery of services or products to the customer exactly when they were promised them. For example, ensuring operations are conducted as scheduled without cancellations.

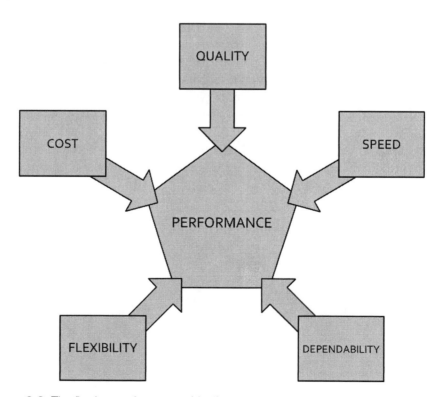

Figure 2.2: The five key performance objectives

Flexibility

Flexibility reflects the ability of the operation to be changed. This change may be providing a new service or product, volume of output or timing of delivery. In cases of epidemics, seasonal changes or crises, hospitals need to be flexible in order to meet demands.

Cost

Cost is an important determinant of performance. This being particularly relevant in healthcare where budgets are often restricted. Operation costs may be considered in three broad categories.

➤ Staff costs.
➤ Resources – equipment, technology, facilities.
➤ Inputs – materials.

Quality

Quality is defined by ensuring things are done correctly. Quality is the most visible part of the operations process. Quality can be characterised according to a number of features, including functionality, appearance, reliability, durability and contact. In a healthcare setting, quality may be defined as the provision of safe, effective, patient-centred, timely, efficient and equitable care. The delivery of optimum quality healthcare should be the primary goal of any medical institution or practitioner.

Service quality has been shown to have a large impact on performance, consumer satisfaction, consumer loyalty and profitability. An understanding of service quality models is therefore crucial in a healthcare setting where there is direct contact with a consumer seeking a service.

Parasuraman (1985) proposed that service quality may be described as a function of differences arising from consumer expectations and perceptions.[2] These result in a gap between expectations and perceptions, hence this model also being referred to as the gap model. Consumer expectations describe what the consumer wants. These expectations are formed from marketing, advertising, word of mouth, prior experiences, and personal needs. Consumer perceptions are formed when they are served during their interactions with the organisation. Five main gaps have been identified that occur during the service process (*see* Figure 2.3).[2] Four of these gaps occur during service provision and are influenced by the management and provider, hence open to change.

Gap 1 represents the difference between the consumers' expectations and the management's perception of those expectations. This primary gap arises when the management does not understand what the consumer expects.

Gap 2 is the management perception – service quality specifications gap. This arises when consumers expect a certain type of service that is not delivered despite the management believing such quality of service exists.

Gap 3 is the service performance gap. This is the difference between service quality specifications and actual service delivery.

Gap 4 is the service delivery – external communications gap. This gap represents whether promises made to consumers are actually delivered by the service.

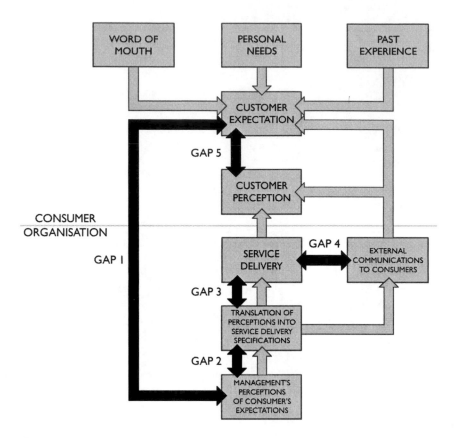

Figure 2.3: Parasuraman consumer expectation-perception gap model [2]

These gaps have a consequential effect on the final gap that is the consumer expectation – perception gap.

Gap 5   represents how consumers perceive the actual service performance in the context of their expectations.

Based on this research the SERVQUAL scale was conceptualised for measuring consumer expectations and perceptions of service quality. Five dimensions of service quality are measured using the SERVQUAL scale. These dimensions are: tangibles; reliability; responsiveness; assurance; and, empathy. Tangibles relate to the appearance of facilities, equipment, and personnel. Reliability is the ability to perform promised services dependably. Responsiveness represents the willingness to help consumers and provision of a prompt service. Assurance is conveyed by providers' ability to communicate in a credible, competent and courteous manner. Empathy relates to understanding consumers and provision of a caring individualised service. SERVQUAL has been used widely in a healthcare setting assessing patient satisfaction and expectations in a variety of services.

Case study

Service quality in NHS hospitals, UK

Youssef *et al.* used the SERVQUAL instrument to measure patients' satisfaction with service quality in West Midlands NHS hospitals, from the moment of referral to discharge. The received 174 responses, which explored the patients' expectations and perceptions of each of the fives dimensions of the SERVQUAL instrument (see below).

Tangibles
• Excellent hospitals would have up-to-date facilities. • Physical facilities at excellent hospitals would be visually attractive. • Hospital staff would be neat in appearance. • Materials associated with the hospital's service would be visually appealing.
Reliability
• Excellent hospitals would provide their services at the time they promise to do so. • When a patient has a problem, excellent hospitals would show a sincere interest in solving it. • Excellent hospitals would carry out services right the first time. • Excellent hospitals would provide error-free documentation. • Hospital staff in excellent hospitals would tell patients exactly when services will be performed.
Responsiveness
• Hospital staff in excellent hospitals would give prompt service to patients. • Hospital staff in excellent hospitals would always be willing to help patients. • Hospital staff in excellent hospitals would never be too busy to respond to patients' requests. • The attitude of hospital staff in excellent hospitals would instill confidence in patients.
Assurance
• Patients would feel secure in receiving medical care at excellent hospitals. • Hospital staff in excellent hospitals would always be courteous with customers. • Hospital staff in excellent hospitals would have the knowledge to answer patients' questions. • Excellent hospitals would be approachable
Empathy
• Excellent hospitals would give patients individual attention. • Excellent hospitals would listen to patients and keep patients informed. • Excellent hospitals would have 24-hour availability. • Excellent hospitals would have the patient's best interest at heart. • Hospital staff of excellent hospitals would understand the specific needs of patients.

Their results revealed that patients' perceptions failed to meet their expectations in all dimensions except tangibles. The survey showed that patients' expectations of service providers are highest for reliability. This was, however, perceived to be the worst feature of the NHS hospitals by all respondents. This study highlights the usefulness of the SERVQUAL instrument in assessing service quality in healthcare.

Employment of methods to improve performance

Having defined the five performance objectives and how to measure them, we must then look at how to improve them. A significant body of research has been undertaken exploring methods of improving quality in healthcare. A number of methods of quality improvement currently being used in healthcare originate from industries such as car manufacturing. We will now explore a number of quality improvement methodologies.

Six Sigma

In the 1980s, Motorola popularised the Six Sigma quality approach. The term is derived from statistics where sigma describes the standard deviation and thus number of defects produced in a process. Defects refer to any compromise of product or service quality, profitability, or customer satisfaction. Six Sigma therefore refers to the point from the mean when measures are required for correction of a process. It is a technique of reducing defect rates by using process improvement, product development and statistical methods.[3,4] Thus a Six Sigma process is one in which 99.99966% of the products or services produced are statistically expected to be free of defects, i.e. 3.4 defects per million! (Can we apply it in medicine? For example, in 1 million carpal tunnel surgeries there should only be 3.4 instances of median nerve damage.) Six Sigma aims to identify the customer's needs and address why there is variation in meeting these needs. The Six Sigma process consists of a number of steps (DMAIC).

➤ **Define** – What is the process purpose and scope?
➤ **Measure** – What is the current process baseline?
➤ **Analyse** – What accounts for errors or loss of quality in the process?
➤ **Improve** – What can we do to improve performance? How can we implement these changes?
➤ **Control** – What difference have we made? What recommendations can be made to sustain improved quality of the process?

The main steps involved in the DMAIC process improvement model are shown below (*see* Figure 2.4).[3]

A number of studies have used Six Sigma in a healthcare setting with successful outcomes. These studies have shown improvements in efficiency, reduced errors, less complaints and increased savings. Examples include implementation of Six Sigma in radiology and pathology departments resulting in significantly improved efficiency and subsequent reduction in costs. The number of studies remains relatively small but there is evidence to suggest potential benefits of Six Sigma.

Case studies

The application of the Six Sigma programme for the quality management of the PACS

The Picture Archiving and Communications System (PACS) is a method of reviewing a patient's radiological investigations via a computer terminal. The system has become an integral part of most hospitals now and any errors or downtime in the system can result in a significant impact on delivery of care. In this study, errors and defects produced by the system in various stages of the process from image acquisition to delivery were identified. This allows for production of a process map and an opportunity to identify areas that can be improved. Based on the statistical significance of the defect and resources required to improve the process measures were instituted. Measures included replacement of machines with frequent errors, improving the memory of existing computers, and staff education programmes. The study found that after six months of implementation of measures, the overall resource requirement was improved by 79%.

Six Sigma in healthcare: lessons learned from a hospital

One of the first healthcare organisations to implement Six Sigma was the Commonwealth Health Corporation, Kentucky in 1998. They reported a 33% improvement in their radiology department throughput and 21.5% reduction in cost per procedure. The result of this at the beginning of 2002 was a saving in excess of $2.5 million. The Thibodaux Regional Medical Center, Louisiana has also implemented a number of Six Sigma projects. These focused on areas such as accounts receivable days, patient safety, hospital acquired infection, medication management and employee satisfaction. They reported savings of more than $475 000 per year following implementation of these programs.

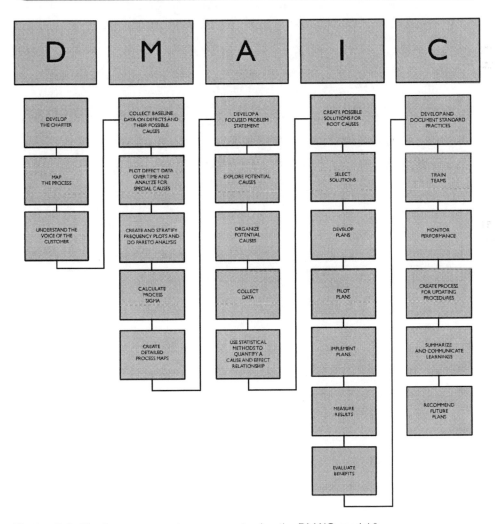

Figure 2.4: Six sigma process improvement using the DMAIC model [3]

Lean

Lean is a method of process improvement developed by Toyota in the 1950s based on work conducted by Taylor and Deming. The concept involves improving the process flow by eliminating waste. Waste may be considered as defects, inappropriate processing, unnecessary inventory, overproduction, waiting delays, unnecessary motion or transportation. A Lean process ensures that the right things are delivered in the right quantities to the right place, at the right time, while minimising waste and being flexible and open to change.[4,5] Lean comprises five main principles.

➤ **Identify customer value** – What do customers consider to be important? In healthcare value can be described as any activity that improves the patient's health.

➤ **Manage value stream** – The value stream is may be considered as the patient journey. We need to identify the processes required to deliver value for patients.

➤ **'Flow' production** – How will materials and information flow through the process? Align healthcare processes to facilitate the smooth flow of patients and information.

➤ **Pull work through the process** – How can we let patients pull the services needed rather than pushing it to them.? This is about providing care on demand and utilising resources at that time.

➤ **Pursue perfection through reducing all forms of waste in the system** – How can processes be optimised? This is the continual development and adjustment of process to achieve the ideal outcomes.

In a clinical setting using lean, an introduction of non-elective trauma patient care pathway in a UK hospital resulted in a significant reduction in mortality and shorter length of stay.[6] Numerous other examples of Lean implementation resulting in improved patient care have been described in the literature.

Case study

Reducing mortality in hip fracture patients

The Bolton Improving Care System group reviewed the care pathway of patients admitted with fractured neck of femur fractures. This patient group had a significantly higher than average mortality rate. The group's work highlighted delays and errors that took place during the patient's journey.

This lead to implementation of changes such as the following.
- A dedicated hip fracture unit.
- Consultant orthogeriatrician and multidisciplinary team input.
- Fast-track transfer from emergency department to ward.
- Re-organisation of theatre to allow for capacity of trauma demand.
- Ward improvements using rapid rehabilitation and early warning scores.
- Listening to experiences of patients and carers in order to improve services.

Following these changes, the group found that there was a significant reduction in mortality, to 15% lower than the national rate. There were also reductions in hospital stay and time taken in theatre.

Lean Six Sigma

Improvement of processes using both Lean and Six Sigma has been shown to be beneficial in healthcare. Benefits reported include improvement in clinical outcomes, process of care, increased throughput, reduced waiting times and medication errors.[7] The main differences between the two methods are summarised in Table 2.1.

Table 2.1: Six Sigma and Lean[4]

	Six Sigma	**Lean**
Theory	Reduce variation	Reduce waste
Application guidelines	Define Measure Analyse Improve Control	Identify value Identify value stream Flow Pull Perfection
Focus	Problem	Flow
Assumptions	A problem exists Figures and numbers are valued System output improves if variation in all processes is reduced	Waste removal will improve performance Many small improvements are better than systems analysis
Primary effect	Uniform process output	Reduced flow time
Secondary effects	Less waste Fast throughput Less inventory Improved quality	Less variation Uniform output Less inventory Improved quality
Criticisms	System interaction not considered Processes improved independently	Statistical or system analysis not valued

The NHS Institute for Innovation and Improvement has proposed a method of process improvement by combining Lean and Six Sigma (*see* Figure 2.5). This Lean Six Sigma method draws on the benefits of both process improvement techniques.

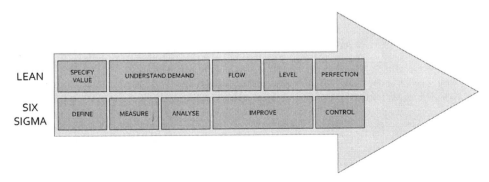

Figure 2.5: Lean Six Sigma [4]

Case study

Quality in trauma care: improving the discharge procedure of patients by means of Lean Six Sigma

A study undertaken in a trauma centre in the Netherlands used Lean Six Sigma to reduce hospital stay. They reviewed admissions to their trauma unit and identified reasons for inappropriate hospital stay such as patients waiting for procedures or investigations, and delays in discharge planning or rehabilitation facilities. The main source of unnecessary hospital stay was found to be patients awaiting a rehabilitation facility or nursing home (49%).

Improvements focused on discharge planning and elimination of all waiting time of the care process. All patients admitted were given an expected date of discharge and organisation of procedures for discharge were put into place at that time. Previously, rehabilitation beds were only arranged postoperatively but now a bed was arranged on the day of admission. At the beginning of the project the average length of stay was 10.4 days. This was reduced to 8.5 days after implementation of improvements. This consequently resulted in an extra 118 admissions, representing a value of €176 000.

Process re-engineering

Business process re-engineering provides a conceptual framework for improving efficiency and effectiveness in a process. Hammer and Champy[8] described that the:

> ... re-engineering of a business process is concerned with fundamentally rethinking and redesigning business processes to obtain dramatic and sustaining improvements in quality, cost, service, lead-times, outcomes, flexibility and innovation.

The basic concept of business process re-engineering has been adapted to the surgical field and become known as surgical process re-engineering.[9]

There are a number of phases involved in surgical process re-engineering (*see* Figure 2.6).

These include the following.

➤ **Identification of the process** – The process may be simply the intra-operative procedure, but may be extended to include the pre- and post-operative periods.
➤ **Process visualisation and analysis** – The current practice is monitored. This may involve time or video analysis. Motion capture analysis has been frequently employed in industry to identify inefficiencies in movements and this can also be applied in surgery.
➤ **Process mapping** – During this phase and the steps of the process are mapped and a process map diagram may be produced. Analysis of the process map allows identification of steps that are deemed unnecessary or may be improved in terms of efficiency and effectiveness.
➤ **Re-design** – Using data from the analysis phase we may then re-design the surgical process.
➤ **Implementation** – The new process is put into practice and assessed using previously employed techniques.
➤ **Evaluation** – The new process is evaluated in terms of previous outcome measures to assess efficiency and effectiveness.

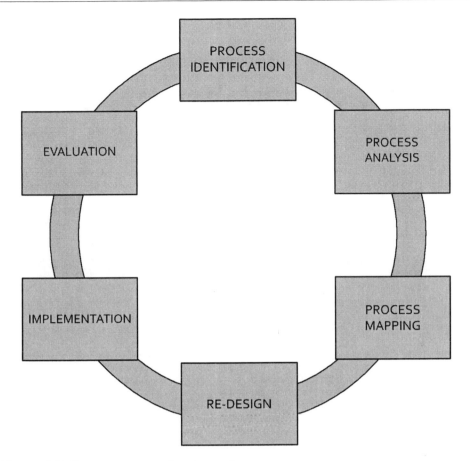

Figure 2.6: The process re-engineering cycle

The framework of surgical process re-engineering is applicable to most medical processes. This may involve analysis of the entire patient journey from referral to treatment or may focus on an individual operative procedure.

In practice, this concept has been applied to carpal tunnel decompression surgery. Caseletto and Rajaratnam[9] reported improved efficiency in this process following the steps outlined above.

Case study

Surgical process re-engineering: carpal tunnel decompression – a model

Carpal tunnel decompression is a common procedure with fairly predictable intra-operative findings. The process was visualised and analysed, producing a detailed process map. The procedure process map comprised 66 steps. These steps were analysed and a number of changes were implemented. An evaluation of five procedures using the re-engineered process was then undertaken. The results revealed a reduction in the number of steps from 66 to 37, and consequent 20% reduction in the time taken to perform the procedure.

Summary

At first glance it may difficult to envisage how a car-manufacturing factory operated by machines may be analogous to a hospital providing care to patients. But through this module, it is hoped the reader can see parallels that are readily transferable to medical practice. At the heart of every consultation or medical intervention, an operations process is taking place. Understanding the theory behind these processes only serves to improve care and service provision. We have seen that manufacturing processes have become highly effective and efficient using the techniques outlined in this module. The reader should appreciate that these can be transferred to their medical practice in order to improve the quality and delivery of care.

Exercises

1 Think about the service that you provide. Consider this according to the five performance objectives. Do you feel that there are any of these that can be improved?
2 You have considered some areas in your service provision that may benefit from process improvement. Devise a plan for process improvement using one of the techniques discussed in this module.
3 Consider a task that is routinely performed with a predictable course of action. Undertake process re-engineering of this task to improve efficiency and effectiveness.

Sample answer for process re-engineering

Process identification
The model employed in this study involved the task of simple suturing by basic surgical trainees. The task given was to perform six simple interrupted sutures in a simulated skin model.

Process visualisation and analysis
The task was captured using digital video for each trainee. The captured footage was then reviewed and key steps identified.

Process mapping
The process was analysed and a process map constructed (*see* Figure 2.7). Analysis of the process map was performed for each trainee and times for each key step recorded.

The pull through and remount steps were those resulting in significant delays in the overall process that could be improved easily. The technical skills were also analysed and advice regarding technique for each trainee formulated.

Re-design
The process was redesigned and areas for improvement identified. The table below summarises the suggested improvements for each step of the process map.

Key step	Improvement
Entry	Needle placement on holder to allow single pass.
Exit	Single-bite suture technique.
Pull through	Suture material handling improvement.
Throws	Knot-tying closer to wound. Reduction in inefficient hand movement.
Cut	Assistant ready in position after second throw.
Reload	Parking of needle whilst performing throws to allow more rapid reloading of needle.

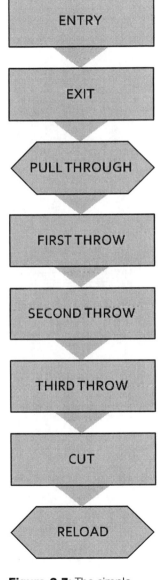

Figure 2.7: The simple suture process map

Implementation

The task was repeated and re-captured. Stopwatch analysis was again performed and the results recorded and compared with the initial performance.

Evaluation

This model has shown significant improvement in the efficiency of the surgical process, with an average improvement of 28.9%. Improvements in the surgical technique and reduced wasted motions were also noted.

References

1   Slack N, Chambers S, Johnston R. *Operations Management*. 4th ed. London: Pearson; 2004.

2   Parasuraman A, Berry L, Zeithaml VA. A conceptual model of service quality and its implications for future research. *Journal of Marketing*. 1985; 49(4): 41–50.

3   Brassard M, Finn L, Ginn D, *et al. The Six Sigma Memory Jogger*. Salem, MA: GOAL/QPC; 2002.

4   Boaden R, Harvey G, Moxham C, *et al. Quality Improvement: theory and practice in healthcare*. Coventry: NHS Institute for Innovation and Improvement; 2008.

5   Jones DT, Mitchell A. *Lean Thinking for the NHS*. NHS Confederation Leading Edge Reports. London: NHS Confederation; 2006.

6   Westwood N, James-Moore M, Cooke M. *Going Lean in the NHS*. Coventry: NHS Institute for Innovation and Improvement; 2007.

7   DelliFraine JL, Langabeer JR, Nembhard IM. Assessing the evidence of Six Sigma and lean in the health care industry. *Quality Management in Health Care*. 2010; **19**: 211–25.

8   Hammer M, Champy J. *Reengineering the Corporation: a manifesto for business revolution*. New York: Harper Collins; 1993.

9   Caseletto JA, Rajaratnam V. Surgical process re-engineering: carpal tunnel decompression – a model. *Hand Surgery*. 2004; 9(1): 19–27.

Case studies

Caseletto JA, Rajaratnam V. Surgical process re-engineering: carpal tunnel decompression – a model. *Hand Surgery*. 2004; 9(1): 19–27.

Kang JO, Kim MH, Hong SE, *et al.* The application of the Six Sigma program for the quality management of the PACS. *American Journal of Roentgenology*. 2005; **185**: 1361–5.

Niemeijer GC, Trip A, Ahaus KTB, *et al.* Quality in trauma care: improving the discharge procedure of patients by means of lean Six Sigma. *Journal of Trauma Injury, Infection and Critical Care*. 2010; **69**: 614–19.

Stacey S, Bhat S, Bolger J. Reducing mortality in hip fracture patients. Available at: www.boltonhospitals.nhs.uk/pdf/reducing_mortality_in_hip_fracture_patients.pdf

Van den Heuvel J, Does RJMM, Verver JPS. Six Sigma in healthcare: lessons learned from a hospital. *International Journal of Six Sigma and Competitive Advantage*. 2005; **1**: 380–8.

Youssef F, Nel D, Bovaird T. Service quality in NHS hospitals. *Journal of Management in Medicine*. 1995; 9: 66–74.

Further reading

➤ Slack N, Chambers S, Johnston R. *Operations Management.* 4th ed. London: Pearson; 2004.

Useful websites

American Society for Quality: http://asq.org/healthcaresixsigma/
NHS Institute for Innovation and Improvement: www.institute.nhs.uk
Heart Improvement Programme: Improving 18 week patient pathways: www.heart.nhs.uk/18weeks/toolsandtechniques/sixsigma.html
Royal Bolton Hospital NHS Foundation Trust – Bolton Improving Care System: www.boltonhospitals.nhs.uk/bics/

Marketing in healthcare

We have all heard of marketing and many consider this simply to mean advertising but there is much more to this term. The American Marketing Association[1] (2007) defined marketing as:

> *Marketing is the activity, set of institutions, and processes for creating, communicating, delivering, and exchanging offerings that have value for customers, clients, partners, and society at large.*

Marketing can, therefore, be defined as the process of ensuring products and services are produced and delivered to the appropriate recipients to satisfy their needs. This process is highly reliant on choosing the right product and then identifying the right target for the product. Throughout this process the organisation must also maintain an advantage over its competitors to ensure consumer needs are met and maintain loyalty.

Marketing and strategy are closely related and it is advisable to read this module in conjunction with the strategy module.

Marketing and healthcare

When exploring marketing in a healthcare setting, it may be useful to consider three different sectors.[2] These sectors are as follows.

➤ **Private** – Within the private healthcare setting, the primary driver is profit for the stakeholders. The organisation uses all strategies to maximise profits and return. Despite this, delivery of care in the community may also be included as part of a hybrid system seen in some developing countries.
➤ **Public** – The public healthcare sector primarily focuses on delivery of good quality healthcare to the public. The Centre for Diseases Control and Prevention (CDC)[3] described health marketing involves '**creating, communicating**, and **delivering** health information and interventions using customer-centered and science-based strategies to protect and promote the health of diverse populations'. They further described health marketing as:

- A multidisciplinary practice that promotes the use of marketing research to educate, motivate and inform the public on health messages.
- An integration of the traditional marketing field with public health research, theory and practice.
- A complex framework that provides guidance for designing health interventions, campaigns, communications and research projects.
- A broad range of strategies and techniques that can be used to create synergy among public health research, communication messages and health behaviours.

➤ **Academic** – of marketing in the academic sector has become increasingly more important. The primary goal here is to attract funding for research. Many institutions previously raised funds for research purely based on word-of-mouth promotion, often detaching themselves from commercialism and entrepreneurism. However, it has become increasingly more apparent that nowadays institutions need to learn to market themselves in order to secure funds and grants.[4]

Despite the differing primary objectives of each of these sectors, the underlying principles of the marketing process remain the same.

Marketing process

We know that there is more to marketing than simply advertising. Kotler[5] described the marketing process as comprising of four stages (*see* Figure 3.1).

➤ Analysis of marketing opportunities.
➤ Selecting target markets.
➤ Developing the marketing mix.
➤ Managing the marketing effort.

We shall now look at each stage in turn and develop an understanding of the basics of the marketing process.

Analysis of marketing opportunities

The first stage is analysis of opportunities and the likelihood of their success. A useful framework for the analysis of the market and the forces driving a product or service comprises the five Cs (*see* Figure 3.2).

➤ **Company** – We need to understand the organisation's structure and positioning relative to competitors, as well as working to identify a firm's core competencies. This involves an analysis of our strengths and weaknesses. Marketing managers need to work with the finance department to analyse the profits or revenues the organisation is generating from various product lines and consumer bases. The organisation may also conduct periodic quality audits to assess the strength of its services and help decide their product and market growth strategy.
➤ **Collaborators** – Collaborators include various suppliers, distributors and other members in the supply chain. This analysis helps identify options of how

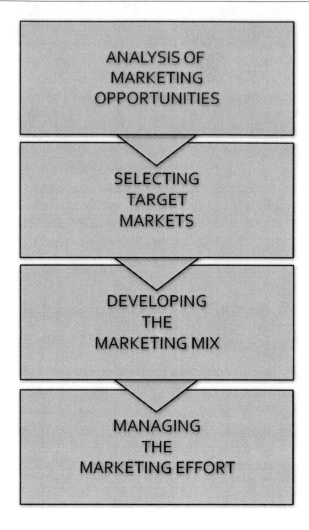

Figure 3.1: The stages of the marketing process

collaboration can improve processes or reduce costs in the production and delivery of a service or product.

➤ **Competitors** – Developing an understanding of how competitors are operating and maintaining their market share or position in the market is very useful. Using SWOT (Strengths, Weaknesses, Opportunities, Threats) analysis described in the strategy module we can identify their strengths and weaknesses. This enables us to exploit opportunities and identify threats. This analysis also allows us to understand their cost structure, pricing, profits, and resources.

➤ **Context** – The context refers to the more global environment in which our organisation is operating. This is based on the PESTEL (Political, Economic, Social, Technological, Environmental, Legal) analysis described in the strategy module. Based on this information decisions regarding investment, growth

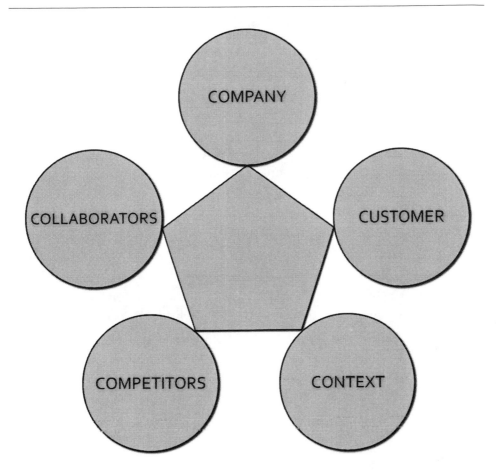

Figure 3.2: The 5Cs framework for analysis of marketing opportunities

strategies, and products can be made in order to meet the needs of the market and its environment.

➤ **Customer** – This involves identifying the customers and breaking them down into focused groups. We need to understand consumer behaviour and spending patterns to help facilitate appropriate methods of attracting them and determining their requirements. This analysis forms the second stage of the marketing process, which is selecting the target markets.

Selecting target markets

This stage involves identification and division of the target market into distinct groups or segments. This process is called market segmentation.[6] Target markets can be divided on the basis of many characteristics including the following.

➤ **Consumer demographic** – Age, gender, income, occupation, education, ethnicity.

➤ **Geographic location** – Region, country, climate.
➤ **Psychographic** – Lifestyle, social class.
➤ **Consumer behaviour** – Brand loyalty, perceived product benefits, purchasing habit (impulsive or informed consumer).

Market segmentation has a number of benefits, which include the following.

➤ Identification of potential gaps in the market.
➤ Identification of growing segments in a slowing or mature market.
➤ Closer matching and tailoring of product or service to consumer needs.
➤ Targeted advertising and distribution.

Once the market segments have been identified an analysis of each is performed to identify the most attractive and hence determine which segments to enter. This process is often referred to as market targeting. Finally, a market position is created in the target by competitive positioning and developing the marketing mix.

Developing the marketing mix

A marketing mix may be defined as a set of controllable, tactical marketing tools that work together to achieve a company's objectives. In 1960, McCarthy[7] described the 4Ps of the marketing mix (*see* Figure 3.3).

➤ Product.
➤ Price.
➤ Place.
➤ Promotion.

Product

The product may be tangible object or intangible service that is offered to the consumer. When considering a product, a number of additional factors must be considered, including the following.

➤ Branding.
➤ Design.
➤ Quality.
➤ Safety.
➤ Support.
➤ Warranty.
➤ Services.
➤ Life cycle.

Product life cycle

The product life cycle defines the stages of a product's development and demise (*see* Figure 3.4).[8] This cycle provides us with an insight into the product's profits and sales during its lifetime. It comprises five stages.

➤ **Development** – During this stage the product requires significant investment for research and development.

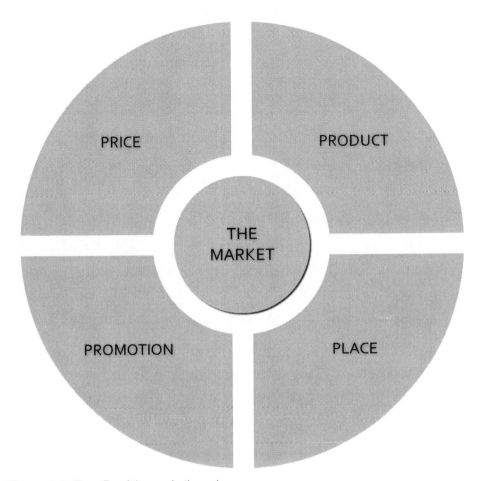

Figure 3.3: The 4Ps of the marketing mix

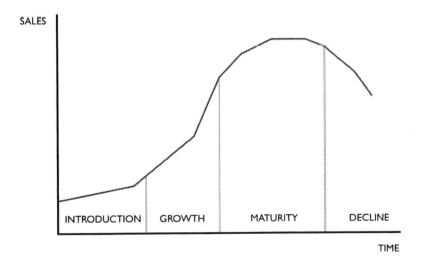

Figure 3.4: The product life cycle [8]

➤ **Introduction** – The product is introduced into the market and the costs of promoting the product far exceeds any sales that are gradually forthcoming.
➤ **Growth** – This is the period of rapid growth in sales and profits.
➤ **Maturity** – The product has become widely accepted and sales slow as the number of new buyers declines. Profits reduce or decline as further investment is required to maintain positioning against competitors.
➤ **Decline** – The demise of the product as both sales and profits decline.

Price

The price of a product or service is an important determinant of survival and profit. Determining the price that a consumer is willing to pay for a product or service relies on a number of factors.

➤ Market share.
➤ Competition.
➤ Demand.
➤ Product identity.
➤ Consumers' perceived value of product.
➤ Special or volume discounts and bundling.
➤ Product life cycle.

The price of a product may change during its life cycle. Initially, at the launch of a product the price may be maintained high since there is no competition, this is pricing strategy is called skimming. Alternatively, in a market where there are already a number of similar products, penetration into the market is required. This involves introducing the product at a low price in order to gain acceptance and market share. The price may then be increased. As we gain economies of scale (producing more at lower costs) and other cost advantages the price may be lowered whilst still maintaining a profit – this is known as sliding on the demand curve. Demand-based pricing is determined by what a consumer is willing to pay. Loss leader pricing occurs at the end of the product life cycle when products are sold below cost to attract consumers to other products made by the company.[6] Kotler has described the Nine Price/Quality Pricing Strategies (*see* Figure 3.5).[5] This provides a useful method of devising pricing strategies based on the price and quality of a product or service.

Place

The place refers to how a product is delivered to a customer. Distribution of a product or service is determined by the following factors.

➤ Distribution channels.
➤ Market coverage.
➤ Order processing.
➤ Storage.
➤ Logistics.

PRICE

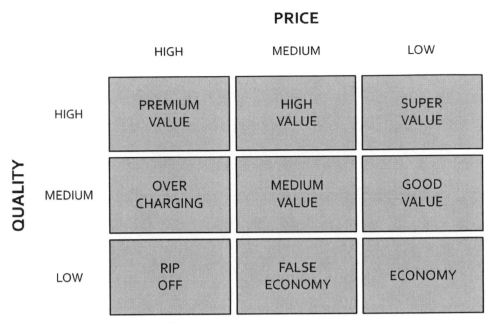

Figure 3.5: Price/Quality Pricing Strategies

Promotion

Promotion relates to communication of a product or service to the marketplace. This message may be relied by a number of means.

➤ Advertising.
➤ Public relations.
➤ Word of mouth.
➤ Point of sale.

In the healthcare sector, word of mouth was the traditional method of promotion. A study by Zavod *et al.* revealed that word-of-mouth referrals were the most important source of predicting which patients would elect to undergo surgery.[9] Kumar *et al.*, based on research from business and industry, produced a categorisation of customers according to the value they bring to a business in terms of sales and referrals.[10] They identify four main types of customer: champions, advocates, affluents and misers. Champions are customers that are good users of the service or purchasers of products but also spread the word about their experiences and encourage referrals. Affluents are customers who buy or spend a good deal but do not spread the word. Conversely, advocates spread the word and promote referrals, but they themselves are not big consumers of the service or product. Finally, misers are customers that neither spend much nor promote much. Using these categories, the companies in their study, targeted each group in a differing manner. The advocates were offered purchasing incentives, affluents given referral incentives, and misers provided with both. In this study, the companies reaped more than a 12-fold return on their marketing investments which was more than double that expected.[10] This helps identify methods of improving our internal marketing and encouraging more champions and advocates.

These days, however, advertising has become increasingly more prevalent. With more competitive markets, a significantly greater proportion of budgets is being spent on advertising in order to attract new potential clients. There are some ethical and regulatory issues to be considered when implementing media advertising. Codes of conduct for media advertising of medical services vary greatly globally. The internet has provided a new platform for marketeers to deliver their efforts to promote services and products. The public sector also utilises significant amounts of health promotion in the form of campaigns to increase awareness of conditions.

People

Although this final P is not part of the original 4Ps, it is one of the most important Ps in healthcare. The people that deliver healthcare are essential to the provision of service. The composition of the teams and their interaction in the care pathway are all essential components of the marketing mix. The interaction of healthcare providers with their clients has an impact on consumer satisfaction, loyalty and future referrals.

Managing the marketing effort

This stage is about the organisation, implementation and control of our marketing plan. The previous stages have analysed all the factors influencing the marketplace, from the external environment down to the product or service. Based on all the analysis, we must produce a strategic plan. This overlaps with the strategy module where we shall look at Porter's five forces, Ansoff's Growth Matrix and three main generic strategies. Having developed the strategic plan we must then implement it.

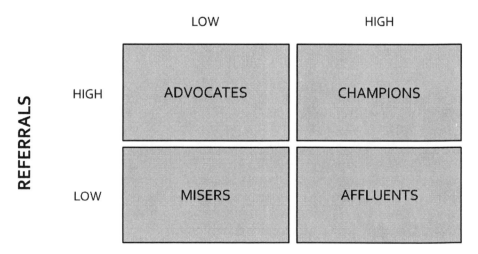

Figure 3.6: Four types of customer according to their value in sales and referrals

The final part of this stage is about controlling our marketing effort. This is a means of monitoring or auditing our strategy to see if we are achieving our desired goals.

Summary

Marketing is relevant to all sectors of healthcare. It can involve setting up health promotion campaigns, raising funds for research or attracting clients to a private practice. This module illustrates the marketing process and highlights important factors in developing a marketing plan, such as the 4Ps. There will invariably be some overlap with strategic management, which we shall now explore in the next module.

Exercises

1   Think about the service you are providing. Who are the main users of your service? What are their demographics? Are there any other groups of users? How can you segment your service provision based on these groups? Can you tailor your service specifically to address the needs of each of these groups?
2   You are considering offering a new product or service. What considerations would you make when deciding on the pricing? Would this pricing change with time?
3   Produce a marketing plan for a new fee for service venture in a healthcare setting of your choice.

Sample answer for a marketing plan

Background

OrthoBase is a new healthcare group that has been set up as a private orthopaedic and trauma hospital. Funding for the venture was derived from shareholders in the company. The main purpose of the company is to address the niche market of orthopaedic and trauma care provision. Emphasis is on care being delivered in the shortest possible time by a team of professionals. This is complemented with an emergency medical service and retrieval system in the form of an in-house ambulance service, air transportation and a 24-hour manned emergency tele-consultation service. The centre also receives patients from outpatient satellite clinics.

Analysis of marketing opportunities

Company

OrthoBase is the only centre of its kind within the country. The site is strategically located in the centre of the country close to a main highway allowing good transport links. The surrounding district has numerous light and small industries that will need healthcare for work-related injuries.

The OrthoBase team comprises 10 consultants who are able to provide a comprehensive and high-quality service. The exclusion of other non-trauma specialties means that the centre is available for the constant provision of trauma care.

The provision of emergency medical services via an ambulance and helicopter service makes OrthoBase a pioneer in this area. A 24-hour emergency medical tele-consultation service provided for by OrthoBase enhances the availability and quality of care provision. The opening up of new satellite clinics will provide further growth for OrthoBase and increase its patient base. The moderate size of the centre also reduces its operating cost favoring a healthy cash flow situation. This will also make it possible for OrthoBase's pricing to be extremely competitive as compared with the other private hospitals.

OrthoBase's main weakness lies in its management skills and financial resources. Since its inception there has been no formal structure and no systems in place. The rapid growth in the first two years without consolidation and financial controls has resulted in severe cash flow problems.

The lack of marketing strategy has also resulted in a lack of accelerated growth in the volume of through put. Also the uniqueness of a niche market and the exclusion of other specialties pose the problem of financial efficiency due to the economies of scale.

Collaborator

OrthoBase has, in association with a specific insurance company, designed a unique healthcare insurance plan called EMTS (Emergency Medical and Trauma Scheme) that will finance this level of healthcare for a nominal premium.

The establishment of a network of associate consultants nationwide by Ortho-Base, has provided the necessary foundation and the first step in the provision of a national medical trauma centre.

Competitors

The bulk of the trauma services available today are via the public hospitals, with their accompanying constraints. They have a satisfactory infrastructure but lack the personnel and dedication to trauma care, thus the quality of care is diluted. There are delays in transit of the patient to these centres and delay in instituting treatment. The level of care in these centres is at a junior staff level. Private hospitals exist; however, there are none purely dedicated to trauma.

Context

Over 150 000 road accidents occur per year, costing $2 billion to the economy. Annual industrial accidents account for 145 000 cases, costing $4 billion. Of these, 45% pertain to the upper limb, with some resulting in permanent disabling injuries.

There are legislative and regulatory considerations when establishing a private healthcare service. Monitoring of services is also undertaken on a regular basis to ensure quality of care and meeting of requirements.

Customers

Our customer base is composed of trauma patients and is discussed in the selecting target markets.

Selecting target markets

OrthoBase offers a dedicated trauma care service, which is a niche market in healthcare. The majority of orthopaedic work consists of trauma and the fact that orthopaedic surgery is a high profit margin specialty allows for good cash generation for profitability. Trauma is mainly the result of road traffic and industrial accidents, and is covered by most insurance policies thus making financing of private care affordable. The location of the various satellites in areas of high industrial growth and sites allows for visibility and timely service and a captive market.

Developing the marketing mix

Product

OrthoBase provides an intangible service of quality dedicated trauma care. The service is provided by 10 consultants with a good track record of safety and expertise in their sector. The centre is well maintained and provides top-quality facilities for patient care and recovery. When assessing the line of services we provide it is useful to consider the different conditions and treatments on offer. For example, burns care in our centre can be very expensive and require prolonged hospital stay resulting in less generated revenue. In contrast, treatment of smaller injuries as day cases generates more revenue. Based on this analysis, we can consolidate our services and remove burns care from our facility.

Price

OrthoBase offers high-quality care at a lower cost compared with other private healthcare providers. Using Kotler's Price/Quality Pricing Strategies, we would be employing high- or medium-value pricing strategies. We have consolidated our line of services offered, which allows us to focus on particular procedures. We can then develop economies of scale by specialising only in these procedures thus driving down our costs.

Place

OrthoBase is centrally located with good transport links and a dedicated air recovery service. The development of satellite clinics helps improve the market catchment area. Tele-medicine also allows cost effective accessibility.

Promotion

Direct advertising of medical services is not permitted in the media. We can increase awareness of our services by improving our relationships with primary care providers and referrers. Undertaking charitable acts and receiving press coverage also raises public awareness of our services.

Managing the marketing effort

Monitoring of returns following implementation of marketing plan provides a useful method of assessing our success. We should also look at other key performance indicators such as hospital stay, patient satisfaction, transport times, and mean length to definitive treatment.

References

1 American Marketing Association. *Definition of marketing*. Available at: www. marketingpower.com/aboutama/pages/definitionofmarketing.aspx (accessed 31 May 2010).
2 Jofre-Bonet M. Health care: private and/or public provision. *European Journal of Political Economy*. 2000; **16**(3): 469–89.
3 Centers for Diseases Control and Prevention. Healthcare marketing. Available at: www.cdc.gov/healthmarketing/ (accessed 31 May 2010).
4 Souba WW, Haluck CA, Menezes MAJ. Marketing strategy: an essential component of business development for academic health centers. *American Journal of Surgery*. 2001; **181**(2): 105–14.
5 Kotler P, Keller KL. *Marketing Management*. Upper Saddle River, NJ: Pearson Education; 2006.
6 Kotler P, Wong V, Saunders J, *et al. Principles of Marketing*. 4th ed. Harlow: Pearson Education; 2005.
7 McCarthy EJ. *Basic Marketing – A Managerial Approach*. Homewood, IL: Irwin; 1960.
8 Levitt T. Exploit the product life cycle. *Harvard Business Review*. 1965; **43**: 81–94.
9 Zavod MB, Adamson PA. Analysis of the efficacy of marketing tools in facial plastic surgery. *Journal of Otolaryngol Head Neck Surgery*. 2008; **37**: 299–308.
10 Kumar V, Petersen A, Leone RP. How valuable is word of mouth? *Harvard Business Review*. 2007; **85**: 139–44.

Further reading

➤ Kotler P, Clarke RN. *Marketing for Health Care Organizations*. Englewood Cliffs, NJ: Prentice-Hall; 1987.

➤ Kotler P, Keller KL. *Marketing Management*. Upper Saddle River, NJ: Pearson Education; 2006.

➤ Kotler P, Wong V, Saunders J, *et al*. *Principles of Marketing*. 4th ed. Harlow: Pearson Education; 2005.

➤ O'Neil JF. Developing, implementing, and sustaining a marketing plan. *American Journal of Orthodontics and Dentofacial Orthopedics*. 2003; **124**(6): 613–14.

➤ Wade T, Seifert P. Marketing the practice. *Seminars in Breast Disease*. 2008; **11**(4): 187–94.

Useful websites

The Charted Institute of Marketing: www.cim.co.uk/resources/
American Marketer's Association: www.marketingpower.com/
Centers for Disease Control and Prevention: www.cdc.gov/healthmarketing/

Strategic management for clinicians

Strategy

A strategy may be defined as a plan to achieve a specific goal. The origins of current business strategy arise from military practice and warfare. Sun Tzu's *The Art of War*, written in the sixth century BC, is one of best-known texts on military strategy.[1] The book has also become a key text in the business world as parallels are readily drawn between the worlds of warfare and business.

Strategy is the process of pursuing a vision and planning how to achieve it.[2] When devising a strategic plan it is therefore useful to consider a number of key stages.

➤ Objective.
➤ Analysis.
➤ Plan.
➤ Implementation.
➤ Evaluation and control.

Objective setting

The first stage in any strategic plan is defining our goal or end-point. What are we trying to achieve and what are our objectives? When defining goals it is useful to use the SMART framework of objectives.

➤ **Specific** – A clear and unambiguous objective
➤ **Measurable** – We must have a measurable outcome for our objective. In business this is frequently a financial outcome. In medicine, disease specific outcomes or mortality are often used as measurable variables.
➤ **Agreed** – The team must be involved and agree to the objective. If there is no support along the whole chain of workers it is unlikely the objective will be successfully achieved.
➤ **Realistic** – Objectives should be realistic and within reach of those involved. Unrealistic outcomes can result in demoralised and demotivated team members, with subsequent failure to achieve the goals.

➤ **Time based** – Setting a deadline for completion of the objective.

Case study

A simple example of a SMART objective may be:

Reduce the number of smokers in a family practice by 50% within the next six months.

Analysis

Sun Tzu in *The Art of War*[1] wrote:

> So it is said that if you know your enemies and know yourself, you can win a hundred battles without a single loss. If you only know yourself, but not your opponent, you may win or may lose. If you know neither yourself nor your enemy, you will always endanger yourself.

This quote highlights the importance of knowing yourself and the environment around you. This is the essence of the analysis stage, which looks internally (yourself) and externally (the environment). In order to undertake effective analysis there some useful methods described to explore ourselves, the in which sector we operate and the more global environment. These methods include:

➤ SWOT
➤ Porter's Five Forces
➤ PESTEL.

SWOT analysis

A SWOT is a method of analysis employed in strategic planning.[3] The analysis explores both the internal focus of the organisation and its external environment. SWOT stands for:

➤ **Strengths** – What are we good at and do better than our competition?
➤ **Weaknesses** – Where are we losing out to competitors?
➤ **Opportunities** – Are there any opportunities arising?
➤ **Threats** – Are there any emerging threats to our organisation?

Identification of these factors then allows us explore relationships between them and how to exploit them. The strategic implications of these relationships are shown in the diagram (*see* Figure 4.1).

Porter's five forces

In 1979, Porter[4] described five major forces that determine the state of competition in a particular industry or sector (*see* Figure 4.2).

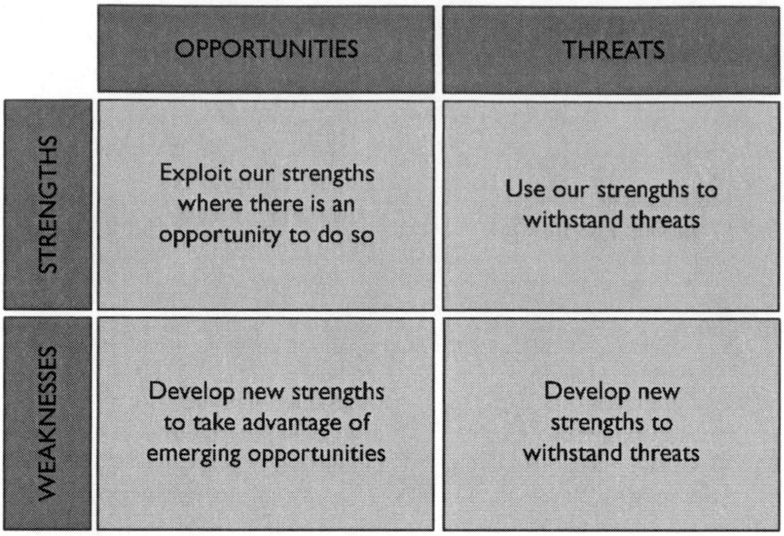

	OPPORTUNITIES	THREATS
STRENGTHS	Exploit our strengths where there is an opportunity to do so	Use our strengths to withstand threats
WEAKNESSES	Develop new strengths to take advantage of emerging opportunities	Develop new strengths to withstand threats

Figure 4.1: SWOT analysis

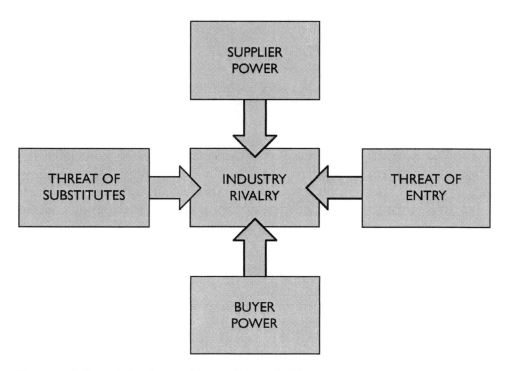

Figure 4.2: Porter's five forces of competitive analysis[4]

These five forces are discussed below.

Threat of entry

New entrants bring with them a threat to existing organisations in that industry or sector. The barriers to entry and reaction of existing organisations determine the size of this threat. There are a number of major sources of barriers to entry, which include the following.

Economies of scale

New entrants when competing against large established organisations could face cost disadvantages and the need to enter on a large scale. Established organisations will have already invested resources into production, marketing, research and distribution. Therefore the cost of producing to a single unit by a large firm will be small.

Product differentiation

Branding and customer loyalty need to be overcome by new entrants. This will often require heavy investment by entrants to attract consumers to their product or services.

Capital requirements

New entrants may need to invest heavily to enter and compete in an industry. These up-front costs required for advertising, research and development can pose a high barrier of entry for new organisations.

Cost disadvantages independent of size

These factors include advantages stemming from patents, access to raw materials, proprietary technology, learning curves, favourable locations and governmental support.

Access to distribution channels

Newcomers face barriers of gaining distribution. Whether its gaining shelf space in a store or costs associated with distribution their product, this barrier can often prevent new entrants from getting off the ground.

Governmental and legal barriers

License requirements or regulated industries limit the number of entrants. Patents, copyrights and other protected intellectual property also restrict newcomers.

Threat of substitutes

Substitutes are alternatives to a product or service offered that fulfil a similar function. The presence of close substitutes means consumers may switch to alternatives if there is an increase in price. This is often seen in a the pharmaceutical industry where closely related medications are often marketed.

Power of suppliers

Suppliers have power over an industry by increasing prices of materials or reducing the quality of their products or services. This in turn impacts the amount of profit made by an organisation. Factors determining a powerful supplier include the following.

➤ **Number of suppliers** – A smaller number of suppliers in comparison with the number of firms it sells to.
➤ **Product differentiation** – If the supplier has a unique or highly differentiated product.
➤ **Switching costs** – Fixed costs associated with changing supplier as a result of need to change equipment, software, etc.
➤ **Threat of forward integration** – There is always a threat that a supplier may integrate into one of its customers thus posing major problems for other customers.
➤ **Nature of industry** – If a particular industry is the primary focus of the supplier then the profits of the supplier will be determined by that industry. Consequently, it is in the interests of the supplier to ensure protection and success of that industry by reasonable pricing, research and development.

Power of buyers

Buyers can also determine the profits of an industry by driving down price, demanding higher quality and playing competitors off one another. The strength of buying power arises from two main factors.

➤ **Buyers' price sensitivity** – If there is a high availability of similar undifferentiated products then buyers can shop around. The buyers' dependence on a product will also determine how much they are willing to pay.
➤ **Relative bargaining power** – The informed customers are better positioned to bargain. The size of the buyer for a product is also important. For example, a health insurance company can purchase healthcare at a lower price than an individual patient.

Competitive rivalry

The intensity of competition amongst rival organisations is dependent on a number of factors.

➤ **Concentration** – The number of competitors determines the level of rivalry. If there is a single company, or monopoly, then there is no competition and the company can decide how much to charge. When there is a small group of companies, or oligopoly, prices are similar. This arises either through collusion or parallel pricing. With increasing number of competitors, there is increasing competition in relation to pricing and price-cutting may be initiated.
➤ **Diversity of organisations** – Similar organisations in terms of objectives, strategies and costs can employ collusive pricing to avoid price competition.
➤ **Differentiation** – If the substitutes are similar then it is more likely that prices from rival companies will be cut in order to increase their sales.
➤ **Exit barriers** – These are the costs associated with leaving an industry. These costs may be specialised equipment, employee reimbursement, or managerial loyalty.

This five forces framework is a very powerful method of analysis that is frequently utilised in industry. The next level of analysis involves looking at the more global environment.

PESTEL

The PESTEL framework provides a method of analysing the macro-environment around an organisation (*see* Figure 4.3).[5] The components of the acronym are as follows.

➤ **Political** – The political factors include specific regulations and policies set out by governments. Government policy has a huge impact on the health of the nation, from funding to workforce issues.
➤ **Economic** – The economic climate influences whether an organisation will pursue certain activities. Issues to be considered include taxation, interest rates and inflation.
➤ **Social** – Social trends are important in planning strategies. The population, for example, is ageing and this should be considered in allocation of resources for older patients. Fashions will also dictate demand for specific procedures such as cosmetic surgery.
➤ **Technological** – Technology is advancing and analysis of our capabilities is important. Research, development and innovation are factors that should be considered in a strategic plan as they can reduce costs and improve quality of care provided.
➤ **Environmental** – Environmental factors include weather and climate change. This can be important in strategy, which may wish to seek environmentally friendly solutions.
➤ **Legal** – Legislation may have an impact on strategic planning. Examples include minimum wage and age and disability discrimination.

Plan

Once we have clearly defined our objectives and analysed our environment, we need to formulate a plan.

Porter's strategies

Porter[6] described three main generic strategies an organisation may develop (*see* Figure 4.4).

➤ **Cost leadership** – The cost leadership strategy is concerned with ensuring a firm delivers a product or service at the lowest possible cost to them. This is achieved by a number of methods, including the following.
  – Improvements in operations processes.
  – Large-scale production and economies of scale – The Boston Consulting Group (BCG) coined the term experience curve. This concept explains the relationship between cost and experience. Their research showed that when the total number of a product made is increased, the cost of production will reduce significantly.

– Technological advances.

– Outsourcing of activities.

➤ **Differentiation** – Differentiation exists when a firm has product or service that offers something unique not provided by its competitors. When establishing a competitive advantage based on differentiation, an emphasis is placed on the following.

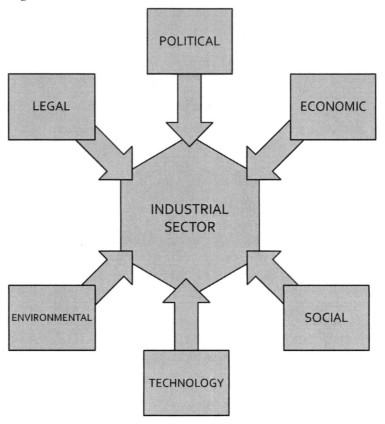

Figure 4.3: PESTEL analysis

SOURCE OF COMPETITIVE ADVANTAGE

	COST	DIFFERENTIATION
WHOLE MARKET	COST ADVANTAGE	DIFFERENTIATION ADVANTAGE
SPECIFIC SEGMENT	FOCUS	

COMPETITIVE SCOPE

Figure 4.4: Porter's generic strategies[6]

- Advertising and branding.
- Design.
- Quality.
- Innovative product or service.
- Research and development.

➤ **Focus** – The focus strategy homes in on a specific market segment and creates either a cost or differentiation advantage for that segment. This can also be referred to as the niche market.

Ansoff product-growth matrix

Ansoff described the 'strategies for diversification' in 1957.[7] This is a useful tool for devising growth strategies for an organisation based on their products or services, and new or existing markets (*see* Figure 4.5).

Based on this matrix, there are four possible growth strategies.

➤ **Market penetration** – This method of growth carries the least risk. Growth occurs by using existing products or services in an existing market. The aim is to attract customers from competitors, achieve new customers or sell more to existing clients.

➤ **Product development** – This method of growth relies on producing a new product or service in an existing market.

➤ **Market development** – This strategy uses existing products or services in new markets. The existing products or services may be targeted at different market segments.

➤ **Diversification** – This strategy carries the highest risk as you are launching new products or services into new markets.

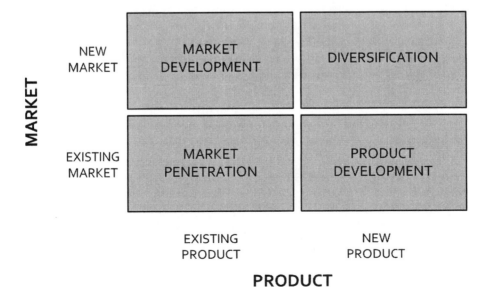

Figure 4.5: Ansoff Product-Market Growth Matrix

Case study

A family physician practice is considering strategies for growth. Using the Ansoff matrix, identify the possible growth strategies.

- **Market penetration** – Attracting more patients involves promotion of our services to the area. This may also attract patients from nearby practices. We may consider developing a practice website or leaflets placed in various locations around the area.
- **Product development** – In our area there is high rate of teenage pregnancy. We may consider providing a sexual health and education service for younger members of our practice.
- **Market development** – We already have a specialised clinic for our older patients offering regular health checks such as blood pressure monitoring. We can offer this same service to the younger male patient group who may not routinely attend the practice.
- **Diversification** – We can consider growth by adding a dispensing pharmacy to the practice.

Implementation

When implementing any plan support from all parts of an organisation or team is required to ensure its success. Implementation of a plan requires input from various management processes. These supporting processes are discussed in other modules and include:

➤ accounting
➤ marketing
➤ operations.

Evaluation and control

The final stage of a strategic plan is evaluation and control. We need to evaluate if our plan has been successful by determining if our defined objectives have been achieved. Control involves further analysis using the methods described above to identify areas for improvement and development in order to maintain a competitive advantage.

Summary

Strategic management and planning is an important process in any organisation. We have seen that a clear definition of our objectives is crucial. Subsequent analysis of the organisation, sector and macro-environment allows us to plan how to achieve our objectives. Once the plans have been implemented, evaluation is required to determine if the objectives have been met. Finally, we need to control our processes and continually analyse them for improvement and maintenance of a competitive advantage (*see* Figure 4.6).

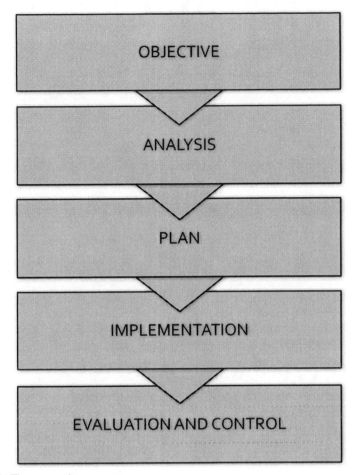

Figure 4.6: The strategic process

Exercises

1 Think of a goal you would like to achieve. Now define that goal using the SMART framework. Does that make the goal more realistic and achievable?

2 Consider your practice. Perform an internal and external analysis of your practice using SWOT and PESTEL. What are your strengths and weaknesses? Have you identified areas for growth and development? What factors could impede your progress?

3 Now consider your goal and how you are going to achieve this? What strategies are you going to employ? How are you going to implement and monitor this?

References

1 Tzu S, Minford J. *The Art of War*. London: Penguin Books; 2009.
2 Grant R. *Contemporary Strategy Analysis*. 5th ed. Oxford: Blackwell Publishing; 2005.
3 Casebeer A. Application of SWOT analysis. *British Journal of Hospital Medicine*. 1993; 49(6): 430–1.
4 Porter ME. How competitive forces shape strategy. *Harvard Business Review*. 1979; 57(2): 137–45.
5 Gillespie A. *Foundations of Economics: additional chapter on business strategy*. Oxford: Oxford University Press. Available at: www.oup.com/uk/orc/bin/9780199296378/01student/additional/page_12.htm (accessed 31 May 2010).
6 Porter ME. *Competitive Strategy: techniques for analyzing industries and competitors*. New York: The Free Press; 1980.
7 Ansoff I. Strategies for diversification. *Harvard Business Review*. 1957; 5: 113–24.

Further reading

➤ Grant R. *Contemporary Strategy Analysis*. 5th ed. Oxford: Blackwell Publishing; 2005.
➤ Hooley G, Saunders J, Piercy N. *Marketing Strategy and Competitive Positioning*. 3rd ed. Harlow: Prentice Hall; 2004.
➤ Swayne LE, Duncan WJ, Ginter PM. *Strategic Management of Health Care Ogranizations*. 5th ed. Oxford: Blackwell Publishing; 2006.

Information technology (IT)

The Information Technology Association of America (ITAA),[1] defines IT as:

> ... the study, design, development, implementation, support or management of computer-based information systems, particularly software applications and computer hardware.

IT deals with the use of electronic computers and software to manipulate, store, protect, process, transmit and retrieve information securely.

IT is now an integral part of medical practice, from patient care to professional development. The modern healthcare organisations throughout the world are now highly reliant on an IT infrastructure for their functioning. Clinicians must therefore be aware of the importance and varying roles of IT in medicine (*see* Figure 5.1), which may be classified as follows.

➤ **Patient care**
  - Electronic medical record (EMR).
  - Imaging.

➤ **Personal development**
  - Research and information.
  - Online education.
  - Scheduling.
  - Social networking.

➤ **Organisational**
  - Hospital intranet.
  - Financial records.
  - Personnel.

We shall explore each of these specific areas and expand on them with examples.

Patient care

In the initial phase of IT in healthcare, its use had been confined mainly to administrative purposes, like the Patient Administration System (PAS) in the NHS. PAS was,

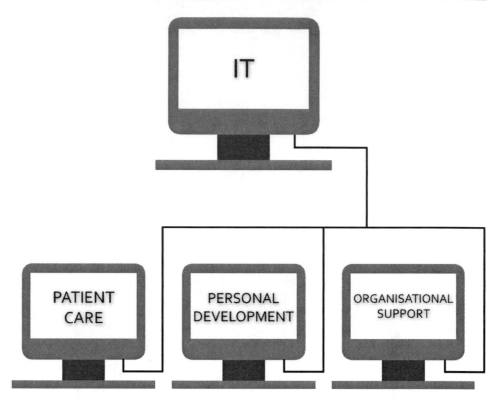

Figure 5.1: IT in healthcare

and continues to be, a computerised system that records patient activity relating to appointments, waiting lists, and case note tracking. It also has the capability to generate reports for local and Department of Health managers detailing waiting times, bed occupancy, and other recordable information for target achievement analysis.

The emergence of new technologies has provided opportunities to digitise further stages in the patient journey. Most hospitals will now possess systems for appointments, investigations, imaging, and record keeping. Integration of these administrative and service components into a unified system has been challenging. This unification leads to the electronic health care record (EHCR). The Medical Records Institute[2] defines five levels of an EHCR.

➤ **The automated medical record** – A paper-based record with some computer-generated documents.
➤ **The computerised medical record (CMR)** – Makes the documents of paper-based records electronically available.
➤ **The electronic medical record (EMR)** – Restructures and optimises the documents of the previous levels ensuring inter-operability of all documentation systems.
➤ **The electronic patient record (EPR)** – A patient-centred record with information from multiple institutions.

➤ **The electronic health record (EHR)** – Adds general health-related information to the EPR that is not necessarily related to a disease.

When moving between hospitals, clinicians will notice significant differences in the software used for patient records and imaging. In order to allow ready exchange of information between the various systems some standards must exist.[3]

➤ **ASTM CCR – Continuity of Care Record** – A patient health summary standard based upon XML, the CCR can be created, read and interpreted by various EHR or EMR systems, allowing easy interoperability between otherwise disparate entities.
➤ **ANSI X12 (EDI)** – Used for transmitting virtually any aspect of patient data. Has become popular in the United States for transmitting billing information.
➤ **CEN – EN13606** – the European standard for the communication of information from EHR systems, and HISA, a services standard for inter-system communication in a clinical information environment.
➤ **DICOM** – A heavily used standard for representing and communicating radiology images and reporting.
➤ **HL7** – HL7 messages are used for interchange between hospital and physician record systems and between EMR systems and practice management systems; HL7 Clinical Document Architecture (CDA) documents are used to communicate documents such as physician notes and other material.
➤ **ISO** – ISO TC215 has defined the EHR, and also produced a technical specification ISO 18308 describing the requirements for EHR architectures.
➤ **Open EHR** – public specifications and implementations for EHR systems and communication, based on a complete separation of software and clinical models.

These systems have primarily been developed for organisations to use and manage their EHCR. The provision of online and software solutions for the storage of personal health information is also becoming readily available. Major companies offering such services include Google and Microsoft. Google Health is a personal health information centralisation service by Google.[4] The service allows Google users to volunteer information such as health conditions, medications, allergies, and lab results. Once entered, Google Health uses the information to provide the user with a merged health record, information on conditions, and possible interactions between drugs, conditions, and allergies. Microsoft's offering is called Health-Vault, a platform to store and maintain health and fitness information.[5]

Imaging

The picture archiving and communications system (PACS) enables images such as X-rays and varying scans to be stored electronically and viewed on displays, creating a near filmless process and improved diagnostic methods.[6] This allows for easy exchange of images between hospitals without the delay and expense of duplicate images and delivery. This has improved patient care in many fields, including neurosurgery where tertiary centres have image links with peripheral hospitals. This allows for scans of patients to be reviewed by the tertiary centre shortly after the investigation is performed at the referring hospital, which minimises unnecessary transfers and provides better delivery of care.

Personal development

Doctors need IT to progress in their personal development. The information overload and the pressures on busy doctors requires them to be able to maximise their potential with IT.

Systems and gadgets help doctors manage time and resources efficiently. The advent of smart phones, such as the iPhone and Blackberry devices, have revolutionised the mobile office and improved efficiency noticeably. Features provided from such devices include cameras, video, web browsing, social networking, push and pull emails, and numerous applications fulfilling virtually every need. Synchronisation of schedules using such devices allows for better time management. It improves one's efficiency, productivity and connectivity at all times, if one so wishes!

Research and information

The internet provides readable accessible information about almost anything direct to the user. Both doctors and patients research and gather information about conditions and treatments using search engines, such as Google. The content of the net is, however, unregulated and therefore there are dangers that the content may be incorrect. Doctors and allied health professionals must be aware of how to obtain accurate and up-to-date information on the internet. An excellent resource to learn how to do online research in medicine for free is available at: www.vts.intute.ac.uk/ tutorial/medicine/

Using search engines, from Google to PubMed, for your research needs requires the understanding of how to search and the use of key search terms.

PubMed provides access to MEDLINE®, the National Library of Medicine's premier bibliographic database containing citations and author abstracts from approximately 5,200 biomedical journals published in the United States and other countries.

MEDLINE uses a controlled vocabulary, meaning that there is a specific set of terms used to describe each article. MeSH is the acronym for 'Medical Subject Headings'. MeSH is the authority list of the vocabulary terms used for subject analysis of biomedical literature at National Library of Medicine. The MeSH controlled vocabulary is a distinctive feature of MEDLINE. It imposes uniformity and consistency to the indexing of biomedical literature. MeSH terms are arranged in a hierarchical categorised manner called MeSH Tree Structures and are updated annually.

For further information on the use of MEDLINE and PubMed visit: www.nlm. nih.gov/bsd/disted/pubmedtutorial/index.html

Intute (www.vts.intute.ac.uk) is a free online service that guides you to the best of the web for education and research. It is run by a national network of university subject specialists who hand-pick relevant websites and organise them under subject headings, with a description of each site.

University and academic websites are also useful research tools; however, they often require active memberships and may be password protected.

In the UK, those working for the NHS can access the NHS resource at www.library.nhs.uk/default.aspx – NHS users can obtain an Athens password from their local hospital library or by visiting: https://register.athensams.net/nhs/nhseng/

The Athens framework of access and identity management products and services that provides staff, students and researchers with easy, single sign-on access to the online resources, databases and journals an institution has subscribed to.

Google Scholar is another resource for searching for academic literature. This service allows users to search and locate articles. Links may be provided for full text versions of certain articles. Google Scholar also uses a ranking system when returning search results that looks at a number of factors, such as who, where and when the article was written

Online education

The internet has provided a new platform for delivery of educational material. Online education can vary from basic websites which provide information to full virtual learning environments. The availability of media such as podcasts and videos also helps to enhance the educational experience. The number of institutions offering online courses is rapidly increasing. Sites also offer continuing professional development programmes that allow users to undertake tests based on information provided and award a certificate on completion.

Scheduling

Time management is an essential skill for all doctors juggling their career, continuous professional development, further education, family, friends, hobbies and other social activities.

Personal information managers (PIMs) are applications that allow you to keep all your information in electronic form. All your appointments, tasks, to do lists, notes, contacts and email messages are stored in a digital and easily accessible form. Numerous applications are available that can be used as PIMs, including iCal, Microsoft Outlook and Google calendar. Some of these may be reliant on specific devices running applications whilst others may be web based. They can often provide synchronisation between various devices. This is useful in allowing administrative or secretarial staff to identify the location of the owner of the schedule.

Social networking

A social network service focuses on enabling virtual communities that allow for the building and reflecting of social networks or social relationships among people. A social network service essentially consists of a representation of each user (often a profile), his/her social links, and a variety of additional services. Most social network services are web based and allow for online communities to be created so that users can interact over the internet, such as by using email, instant messaging and bulletin board services. Such services include blogs, Facebook, Bebo, Twitter and LinkedIn.

Blogs

Blogs are regular entries of commentary, descriptions of events, or other material such as graphics or video.[7] Some people use them as online diaries whilst some medical practitioners have now discovered the usefulness of blogs in relying information to patients. Visitors are allowed to leave comments relating to entries thus allowing interaction with the writer of the blog.

Facebook

Facebook was founded in February 2004 and serves as a social networking platform. Users create a personal profile and then develop a network of friends, family and colleagues. The platform allows users to share photographs, videos, and forthcoming events. Interaction between users using standard messaging and instant online chat are also available. The site currently has over 500 million active users worldwide.[8]

Twitter

Twitter is a social networking microblogging platform that was created in 2006. It allows users to create a profile and create up to 140-character messages, called tweets, that are displayed on their profile. Users can 'follow' other individuals and receive their tweets on their own profile page. The site now has over 100 million registered users, and continues to grow.[9]

Social networking is the new medium of communication across the internet. It appears all ages and professions are embracing the concept of social networking. Now, healthcare needs to also embrace this method of communication.

> The social-networking revolution is coming to health care, at the same time that new Internet technologies and software programs are making it easier than ever for consumers to find timely, personalised health information online.[10]

> It easy to imagine that the combination of both trends — Personal Health Records combined with social networking, what I have called 'PHR 2.0' — may lead to a powerful new generation of health applications, where people share parts of their electronic health records with other consumers and 'crowd source' the collective wisdom of other patients and professionals.[11]

Doctors may use social media to seek out clinical information and opinions and discuss medical points of view with other doctors; to increase their professional exposure among colleagues and the general community; or for purely social reasons – to stay in touch with family and friends.

But beware, there are dangers – a study published in the *Journal of the American Medical Association* in September 2009 stated that 60% of US medical schools reported incidents of students posting inappropriate or unprofessional content on blogs, social networking sites or other places on the internet.[12]

Organisational

At an organisational level, IT provides the backbone for many administrative tasks. IT systems are an integral part of staff management, from human resources to payroll. Finance and accounting rely heavily on IT support for their functioning. There are specific applications relating to specific tasks and departments but these are beyond the scope of this text.

Summary

IT is analogous to the central nervous system, which provides continuous communication of information between all major organ systems within the body. We have seen that IT is important in all aspect of healthcare, from the patient to the clinician to the organisation as a whole.

Exercises

1 Think about all of the IT that you use at work. What applications do you use? How do you think it was done before IT? Can you think of ways of further improving IT systems to provide more efficient and effective patient care?
2 Some are of the opinion that the use of technology will create a distance between clinicians and their patients. If so, what steps could clinicians take to mitigate this?
3 Consider the use of social media networking. Do you feel this may have a place in patient care? Can you think of ways such applications may enhance the overall effectiveness of your practice?

References

1   Wikipedia. Information Technology. Available at: http://en.wikipedia.org/wiki/Information_technology (accessed 31 May 2010).
2   Waegemann CP. The five levels of electronic health records. *MD Comput.* 1996; **13**(3): 199–203.
3   Wikipedia. Electronic Health Record. Available at: http://en.wikipedia.org/wiki/Electronic_health_record (accessed 31 May 2010).
4   Google. Google Health. Available at: www.google.com/health/ (accessed 31 May 2010).
5   Microsoft. Health Vault. Available at: www.healthvault.com/ (accessed 31 May 2010).
6   NHS. Picture Archiving and Communications System. Available at: www.connectingforhealth.nhs.uk/systemsandservices/pacs (accessed 31 May 2010).
7   Wikipedia. Blog. Available at: http://en.wikipedia.org/wiki/Blog (accessed 31 May 2010).
8   Facebook. Facebook Statistics. Available at: www.facebook.com/?ref=logo#!/press/info.php?statistics (accessed 31 May 2010).
9   Wikipedia. Twitter. Available at: http://en.wikipedia.org/wiki/Twitter (accessed 31 May 2010).
10 Landro L. The Informed Patient: social networking comes to healthcare. *Wall Street Journal*; December 2006. Available at: http://online.wsj.com/article/SB116717686202159961.html (accessed 31 May 2010).
11 Eysenbach G. Medicine 2.0: social networking, collaboration, participation, apomediation, and openness. *Journal of Medical Internet Research.* 2008; **10**(3): e22.
12 Chretien K, Greysen SR, Chretien JP, *et al.* Online posting of unprofessional content by medical students. *Journal of the American Medical Association.* 2009; **302**: 1309–15.

Further reading

➤   Wager KA, Lee FW, Glaser JP. *Managing Health Care Information Systems.* San Francisco: John Wiley and Sons; 2005.

Useful websites

NHS Connecting for Health: www.connectingforhealth.nhs.uk/
FaceBook: www.facebook.com
LinkedIn: www.linkedin.com
Twitter: www.twitter.com

Human resource management

The most important component of any healthcare service is the personnel that deliver the service. The latest figures reveal that the UK healthcare service employs over 1.2 million people in the hospital and community health service.[1] Strategic human resource management (SHRM) encompasses numerous activities related to the management of these employees, which include the following.

➤ **Requirements** – Workforce planning.
➤ **Recruitment**.
➤ **Rewards**.
➤ **Retention**.
➤ **Relationships** – Leadership and teamwork.
➤ **Training and development**.
➤ **Appraisal** – Performance management.

In this module we shall explore how to define our employee requirements and how to recruit and retain them. The following modules will look at relationships amongst staff using leadership and teamwork. We shall also see how employees should be trained and appraised.

Strategic human resource management

We have already seen that strategy involves developing a plan in order to achieve a goal. SHRM may be considered as managing our human resources so that they are aligned with the attainment of the long-term organisational goal.[2] This process encompasses many activities that we have already alluded to. We shall now see how to determine the requirements of our workforce, and recruit and retain them.

Requirements

Identification of the staffing requirements of an organisation is the first stage in the human resources planning process. In order to make an assessment of the requirements a number of questions must be addressed.

➤ What is the organisation's vision?
➤ What are the strategic plans for the organisation?

➤ What are the expected staff requirements to fulfil these strategies? Workforce planning addresses this question.

Workforce planning

Workforce planning has been described as 'getting the right people with the right skills and competences in the right place at the right time'.[3] Workforce planning relates to the designing, development and delivery of the workforce. A plan can vary from a simple on call rota to a national plan of staff required to provide a service.

Workforce planning is important in a healthcare setting for many reasons, including the following.

➤ To ensure adequate staff for service provision.
➤ To enable an organisation to respond to targets and governmental policies.
➤ To encourage teamwork between service providers.
➤ To educate and train staff appropriately.
➤ To enhance patient care by delivery of an efficient and effective service.

There are five main strategies that are used in workforce planning.[4]

➤ **Population-based estimating** – This method defines ratios of professionals to population. It is a useful method when considering larger health service organisations such as the NHS.
➤ **Benchmarking** – This method considers existing ratios but also takes into account efficiency of the ratios.
➤ **Needs-based assessment** – This matches the workforce to the healthcare needs of the population in question.
➤ **Demand-based assessment** – This method considers the demand for healthcare professionals. For example, an increase in the elderly population means there will be demand for more elderly care physicians.
➤ **Training-output estimating** – This determines the supply of practitioners based on the anticipated number of graduates.

These different strategies help identify our requirements but we must consider a number of other factors.

➤ **Organisation** – Does the organisational culture allow us to implement these changes? Will the change in workforce affect the organisation?
➤ **Resources** – Do we have the resources to employ the staff required? What impact will the change in the workforce have on existing resource allocation?
➤ **Training** – Do we the facilities to train the workforce to perform their roles adequately? Do we need to train the existing workforce to undertake new roles as a consequence of changes?
➤ **Existing workforce** – What impact will there be on the current workforce? Will there be some employees who will not accept changes?
➤ **Turnover** – Do we have a high staff turnover? Why is this? How can we retain our employees?
➤ **Performance** – Are the employees achieving their targets? How are we going to measure performance after the changes in workforce take place?

Recruitment

We have seen some methods and factors in determining the workforce required to offer a service. We must now recruit the appropriate staff for the positions. The first step in recruitment should be to define the job or position clearly.

Job design

Job design may be considered as the organising of tasks, duties, and responsibilities into a productive unit of work.[2] The design of a job has major implications on the overall performance, satisfaction and health of an employee. The definition of a job can be formulated using the job description.

Job description

➤ **Title** – What is the title given to the position?
➤ **Objective** – What are the objectives of the position?
➤ **Description** – What are the tasks and duties to be performed by the jobholder?
➤ **Role** – What is the primary role in the organisation? Are there any additional roles, such as being a mentor, which the position entails?
➤ **Interactions** – What is the organisational structure and how is the position related to other organisational workers? What are the interactions of this position with superiors and subordinates? Will the position be a part of a team?
➤ **Specifications** – What are the knowledge, skills and attributes that person must possess? Are there any essential qualifications? What are desirable qualities for the position?

We can see this job description helps us identify the person who would be best suited for the position in question. This also forms a good basis for an advertising description for a position.

Case study

An example of an advert for a consultant post in dermatology

Substantive Consultant Post in Dermatology with a Specialist Interest in Skin Oncology

An opportunity to maintain and improve hospital and community based care of patients with skin diseases. The successful candidate will join a team of 10 consultants serving the population of central London.

Duties include provision of general dermatology services and a specialised skin oncology service. The contractual commitment will comprise eight programmed activities dedicated to clinical work and two to teaching and continuing professional development. Clinical commitments will include outpatient clinics, ward referrals and minor procedures lists.

The position will also entail chairing the specialist skin oncology multidisciplinary team. This involves interaction with other hospital services such as oncology, histology, radiology, and plastic surgery.

The successful candidate will be a Member of the Royal College of Physicians or equivalent. They should have also completed higher specialist training or equivalent in dermatology. Desirable requirements include a higher degree and management experience.

For further information and enquiries please contact *********.

Recruitment process

We have clearly defined our position and the next stage in the human resource process involves the recruitment and selection of individuals. The recruitment process involves a number of stages (*see* Figure 6.1).

➤ **Advertising** – This step involves promoting the position vacancy to the appropriate audience. This could range from placing a notice on the hospital notice board or intranet to an international advert in a journal.

➤ **Short-listing** – The specifications in the job description allow us to form essential and desirable criteria for short-listing candidates. This process should be as objective as possible to ensure fairness in the selection of interviewees.

➤ **Interviewing** – The interview can vary from a small informal panel to a multistage process involving proficiency tests.

➤ **Ranking** – The interviewees are next ranked according to their performance and credentials.

➤ **Referencing** – This involves collection of character and professional references from previous employers or colleagues.

➤ **Hiring** – This is the offer of the position to the successful candidate, and subsequent administration including contracts.

Reward management

This aspect of human resources concentrates on the pay and associated benefits gained from achieving objectives. There are two main types of reward.

➤ **Fixed levels of pay** – These are regular salaries paid to employees that are dependent on their position. Incremental increases in pay may be experienced with promotions or annually with increasing seniority.

➤ **Reward linked to performance** – This form of pay is related to the performance of an employee in achieving objectives, from a bonus for securing a major business deal to a tip received from providing service in a restaurant.

(*See* Module 9: Managing clinicians' performance.)

Retention

An understanding of job satisfaction is very important when considering staff retention. Researchers have shown that, at an organisational level, more satisfied employees tend to be more productive. Studies also report a consistent negative relationship between job satisfaction and absenteeism. Satisfaction is also negatively related to turnover, this relationship being stronger than that for absenteeism.[5]

Maslow described the hierarchy of needs, in which five needs exist: physiological, safety, social, esteem, and self-actualisation (*see* Figure 6.2).[6] These are intrinsic needs for that individual. Based on the work of Maslow, researchers have often described job satisfaction in terms of achievement of these needs. The higher the need, the more motivated the individual will be to achieve it.

Herzberg proposed the two-factor theory, or motivation-hygiene theory, where factors leading to job satisfaction are distinct and separate from those that result in job dissatisfaction (*see* Figure 6.3).[7] Factors resulting in satisfaction, described as motivators, were recognition, responsibility, achievement and promotional and personal growth opportunities. These are characteristics that individuals find intrinsically rewarding. Extrinsic factors, described as hygiene factors, resulting in dissatisfaction include quality of supervision, pay, company policies, physical working conditions, relationships with others and job security.[5,7]

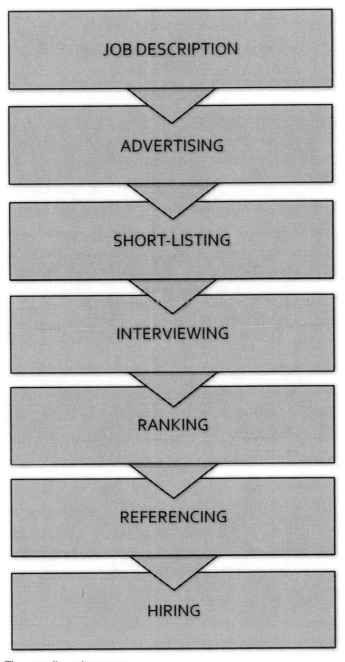

Figure 6.1: The recruitment process

SELF
ACTUALISATION
ESTEEM
SOCIAL
SAFETY
PHYSIOLOGICAL

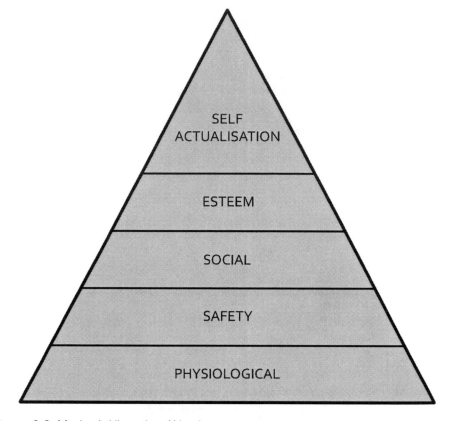

Figure 6.2: Maslow's Hierarchy of Needs

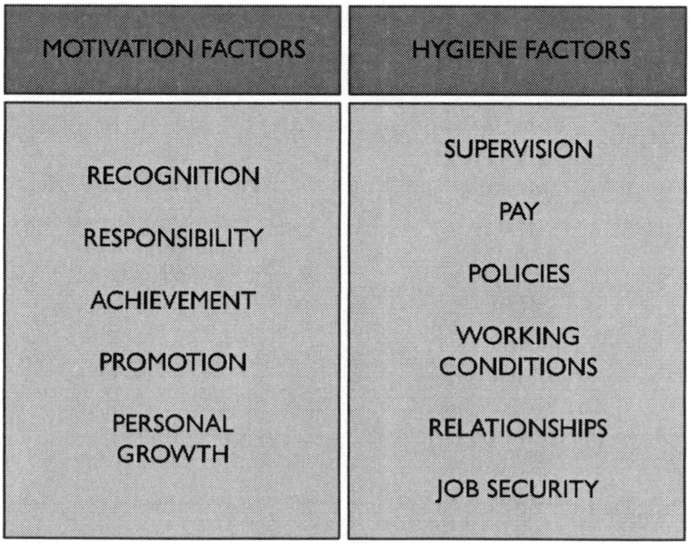

MOTIVATION FACTORS
HYGIENE FACTORS
RECOGNITION
RESPONSIBILITY
ACHIEVEMENT
PROMOTION
PERSONAL GROWTH
SUPERVISION
PAY
POLICIES
WORKING CONDITIONS
RELATIONSHIPS
JOB SECURITY

Figure 6.3: Herzberg's Motivation-Hygiene Theory

Locke identified four factors conducive to high levels of employee satisfaction: mentally challenging work, equitable rewards, supportive working conditions and supportive colleagues.[8]

We have seen the importance of job satisfaction on staff retention and some of the factors influencing satisfaction. Here are some additional factors that may increase satisfaction when designing a job.[2]

➤ **Job enlargement** – Expanding the number of different tasks performed by broadening the scope of the job.

➤ **Job enrichment** – Give employees responsibility for the planning, organisation, control and evaluation of the job. This empowers them and gives them a sense of responsibility.

➤ **Job rotation** – Move people around to cover different jobs thus disrupting the repetitive and monotonous nature of some jobs.

➤ **Variety** – The more variable the skills involved in performing a job, the more meaningful and rewarding it is likely to be.

➤ **Task significance** – The importance and impact a job has on others. Therefore, a doctor helping a patient and their family is likely to find the task meaningful and satisfying.

➤ **Autonomy** – Giving someone more freedom and autonomy gives increased job enrichment.

➤ **Feedback** – It is important to provide feedback to employees. This can help acknowledge and reward good performance, and guide poor performing employees.

Case study

Factors influencing job satisfaction amongst plastic surgical trainees: experience from a regional unit in the United Kingdom

A survey of plastic surgery trainees from a regional unit was undertaken using a validated job satisfaction questionnaire. The survey identified facets of their job that resulted in satisfaction. The nine facets examined were: pay; promotion; supervision; benefits; recognition; policies; co-workers; nature of work; and communication within the organisation.

The results revealed the highest satisfaction from supervision, nature of work and co-workers. Trainees were least satisfied by the working conditions, benefits, and communication within the organisation.

This survey highlights factors that influence job satisfaction in this group of trainees. Using this information, changes can be made in order to improve facets with low satisfaction rates. This may result in higher performance and productivity and lower turnover and absenteeism.

Summary

Arguably the most important component of any healthcare organisation is the providers of the service. An understanding of workforce planning is important in determining service provision. We have reviewed how to describe a job and use this description in the recruitment process. More importantly, we have explored factors that make employees gain satisfaction from their jobs. This in turn enables us to improve productivity and reduce staff turnover and absenteeism. We shall now explore relationships and interactions between leaders, employees and teams.

Exercises

1 Think about your organisational goal. Consider the workforce required to achieve this goal. How can you plan and rationalise this workforce?
2 Consider your current job. Now write a description of your job using the guidelines discussed in this module.
3 Think about your current job. What do you enjoy about your job? What do you dislike about it? Do you feel satisfied? What things can you think of that may improve your job satisfaction?

References

1 NHS. The Health and Social Care Information Centre. *Monthly NHS Hospital and Community Health Service (HCHS) Workforce Statistics in England.* NHS; June 2010. Available at: www.ic.nhs.uk/pubs/provisionalmonthlyhchsworkforce (accessed 30 June 2010).
2 Mathis RL, Jackson JH. *Human Resource Management.* 13th ed. Mason, OH: South-Western Cengage Learning; 2009.
3 NHS. *Skills for Health – Workforce Projects Team: introduction to workforce planning.* NHS; June 2010. Available at: www.healthcareworkforce.nhs.uk/resources/latest_resources/ introduction_to_workforce_planning.html (accessed 30 June 2010).
4 Fried BJ, Fottler MD. *Human Resources in Healthcare: Managing for Success.* 3rd ed. Chicago, IL: Health Administration Press; 2008.
5 Robbins SP. *Organizational Behaviour.* 10th ed. Upper Saddle River, NJ: Prentice Hall; 2003.
6 Maslow A. *Motivation and Personality.* New York: Harper and Row; 1954.
7 Herzberg F, Mausner B. *The Motivation to Work.* 2nd ed. New York: Wiley; 1959.
8 Locke EA. *The nature and causes of job satisfaction.* In: Dunnette MD, editor. *Handbook of Industrial and Organizational Psychology.* Chicago. IL: Rand McNally, 1976; 1297–349.

Case studies

Nassab R. Factors influencing job satisfaction amongst plastic surgical trainees: experience from a regional unit in the United Kingdom. *European Journal of Plastic Surgery.* 2008; **31**: 55–8.

Further reading

➤ Fried BJ, Fottler MD. *Human Resources in Healthcare: Managing for Success.* 3rd ed. Chicago, IL: Health Administration Press; 2008.
➤ Mathis RL, Jackson JH. *Human Resource Management.* 13th ed. Mason: South-Western Cengage Learning; 2009.
➤ Robbins SP. *Organizational Behaviour.* 10th edn. Upper Saddle River, NJ: Prentice Hall; 2003.

Useful websites

The NHS Information Centre – Workforce: www.ic.nhs.uk/workforce
Healthcare Workforce Portal: www.healthcareworkforce.nhs.uk

The clinical team

The clinical team may be defined as a group of clinicians working collectively for the common goal of improving the patient outcome from a clinical episode. A team approach is becoming the norm in medicine, with many conditions now being managed by multidisciplinary teams. The benefits realised include a holistic approach to patient care incorporating a wealth of experience and knowledge from specialists in their fields.

When considering an individual patient, the core team involved in the provision and delivery of care to that patient may be called the strategic clinical unit (SCU). The centre and focus of this team should always be the patient. Within the organisation exist many other teams who complement and support the SCU to achieve its objectives and goals (*see* Figure 7.1).

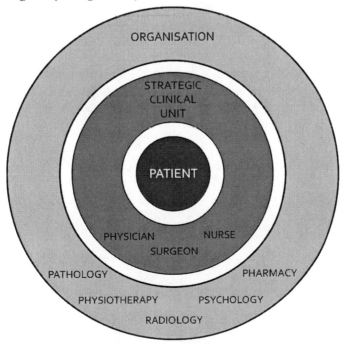

Figure 7.1: The interaction of the strategic clinical unit with the patient and organisation

Anatomy of a team

The anatomy of a team relates to its composition and should ideally consist of members with highly different skill sets that meet the patient's needs both in the immediate and the long term. Teams whose members are more homogeneous tend to be more cohesive but lack the benefits of the diverse skill set. The more heterogeneous team composition will have increased potential for creativity, but greater differences in perspective that can result in greater potential for conflict.

Clinic teams must be dynamic to cater for the changing needs of the situation and patient. Thus the team is ever evolving and changing in composition, functions and hierarchy in tandem with the needs of the situation.

Teams may be formal or informal. Formal teams arise as a consequence of the structure of an organisation, such as a medical team comprising of a consultant and their junior staff. Informal groups are formed when alliances are required to achieve a goal, but they are not structurally or organisationally determined. In the clinical setting one may also classify two types of team depending on the needs:

Independent teams (surgeons operating)

These function on their own and their performance is not dependent on the performance of another member. They tend to perform the same clinical processes. They may be able to help each other by offering opinion or training opportunity, by providing support, or by helping when clinical work becomes busy.

Managing this team requires more intellectual, job-related training and process improvement. Surgical process re-engineering will be a useful tool to help manage this group to improve performance.

Interdependent teams (the surgical team)

Here no significant task can be accomplished without the help of any of the team members. The team members typically specialise in different tasks (anaesthetics, nursing, scrub assistants, runners). The success of every individual is inextricably bound to the success of the whole team.

Managing this team requires an approach where members benefits from getting to know the other team members socially, from developing trust in each other, and being acknowledged and achieving incentives for the desirable collective outcomes.

The best way to start improving the functioning of an independent team is often a single question, 'What does everyone need to do a better job?'

The physiology of the clinical team

Tuckman[1] described the classic team development model, which identified five stages in the progression of building a team (*see* Figure 7.2).

Forming stage

In this initial phase there is a high dependence on a leader for guidance and direction. Often the doctor in an inter-professional team or the most senior member by default takes leadership. There will be role ambiguity among members at this stage and in a new situation the leader must be prepared to define team's purpose, objectives and external relationships.

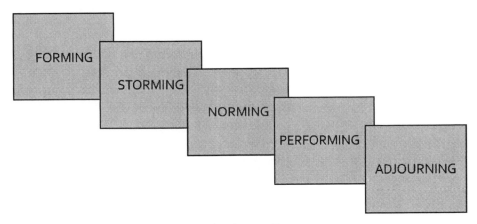

Figure 7.2: Tuckman's stages of team development[1]

Storming stage

The storming stage consists of intra-group conflict. The members accept a group is forming but there is resistance as to the constraints that are placed on individuals. There also exists conflict over the hierarchy of the team and competition for power. This is an important stage in developing a common set of values, beliefs and goals. The emergence of a leader needs to occur to ensure the members understand their goals and roles clearly. Poulton *et al.* showed that clarity of and commitments to team objectives were pivotal in predicting the overall effectiveness of the primary healthcare team. The team also needs to avoid becoming distracted by relationships and emotional issues. This can occur in emotionally charged situations, such as transplant teams, that need special attention.

Norming stage

At this stage cohesiveness and close relationships between members are formed. Once this has occurred team members begin to conform to the norms – these being unwritten behaviours and rules, which are generally accepted by all members of the team. The norms may be considered as the culture and working style of the group. Shared responsibility among members is essential. There is acceptance by the members of the leader and it is at this stage that team-building social activities help to strengthen the members.

Performing stage

This stage is when the team is up and running and undertaking the tasks at hand. At this stage the members are aware of their responsibilities, shared goals and objectives. They are all able to function with independence, with each member understanding their tasks and the overall desired outcomes. The leader needs to delegate his/her duties at this stage and allow for team member empowerment, which is crucial. The quicker a team can reach this stage the more efficient the delivery of its processes and the greater benefit for the patient.

Adjourning stage

This final stage arises when teams are temporary and formed for specific tasks or projects. This final stage arises when the time has come for the team to disband.

It is useful at this stage to reflect on any learning experience and note for future use. In some teams this can be a formal de brief and part of reflective clinical practice.

This is a useful model in understanding team formation. There are, however, other factors that influence how teams form not considered in this model. One of the major factors is the context in which a team is formed. An example would include a resuscitation team that is formed rapidly at a time of emergency. In this context, the members of the team may not necessarily know each other but they know their defined role in the given situation and hence the team is immediately effective. In this example, team members follow roles and protocols laid out in courses such as Advanced Life Support.

Team roles

Belbin[2] defined team roles as 'a tendency to behave, contribute and interrelate with others in a particular way.' The members will each have strengths and allowable weaknesses contributing to completion of a task. Nine different roles individuals play within a team were identified and these are summarised in the table below (*see* Table 7.1).

Table 7.1: Belbin Team Roles[2]

Team role	Contribution	Allowable weakness
Plant	Creative, imaginative, unorthodox. Solves difficult problems.	Ignores incidentals. Too preoccupied to communicate effectively.
Resource investigator	Extrovert, enthusiastic, communicative. Develops contacts.	Over-optimistic. Loses interest once initial enthusiasm has passed.
Co-ordinator	Mature, confident, a good chairperson. Clarifies goals, promotes decision-making, delegates well.	Can be seen as manipulative. Offloads personal work.
Shaper	Challenging, dynamic, thrives on pressure. The drive and courage to overcome obstacles.	Prone to provocation. Offends people's feelings.
Monitor evaluator	Sober, strategic and discerning. Sees all options. Judges accurately.	Lacks drive and ability to inspire others.
Teamworker	Co-operative, mild, perceptive and diplomatic. Listens, builds, averts friction.	Indecisive in crunch situations.
Implementer	Disciplined, reliable, conservative and efficient. Turns ideas into practical actions.	Somewhat inflexible. Slow to respond to new possibilities.

Complete finisher	Painstaking, conscientious, anxious. Searches out errors and omissions. Delivers on time.	Inclined to worry duly. Reluctant to delegate.
Specialist	Single-minded, self-starting, dedicated. Provides knowledge and skills in rare supply.	Contributes on only a narrow front. Dwells on technicalities.

This provides a method of identifying, by use of the Belbin Self-Perception Inventory, the behaviour of individuals within a team.[2]

Building effective teams

We have seen how teams come together, their composition and classification. The development of an effective team is, however, the most important aspect of fulfilling and completing the task at hand. Extensive research has been conducted investigating factors for the formation of effective teams. These factors include the following.

➤ There should be clear team goals with in-built performance feedback.
➤ Effective leadership of the team should be present.
➤ Individuals should feel they are important to the fate of the team.
➤ Individuals should have intrinsically interesting tasks to perform.
➤ Training to learn knowledge and skills in order to perform tasks effectively should be readily available.
➤ Individual contributions should be indispensable, unique, and evaluated against a standard.
➤ There should be good communication between all members of the team.

Team effectiveness model

Once a team forms and becomes effective, continual improvement must be undertaken. The team effectiveness model, produced by the University of Victoria, Canada, identifies five main areas of improvement that should be undertaken by teams to ensure continual improvement (*see* Figure 7.3).[3]

➤ **Goals** – The team must have well-defined and visionary goals that they aspire to.
➤ **Roles** – Clear roles and responsibilities must be given.
➤ **Procedures** – Clear procedures on how the team members can interact and work with each one another.
➤ **Relationships** – How the team members behave and get on with each other.
➤ **Leadership** – Strong leadership supporting their team members to achieve success in obtaining the given goals.

Team dynamics

The interaction between team members is crucial for successful completion of tasks. The main interactions between members include delegation and conflict.

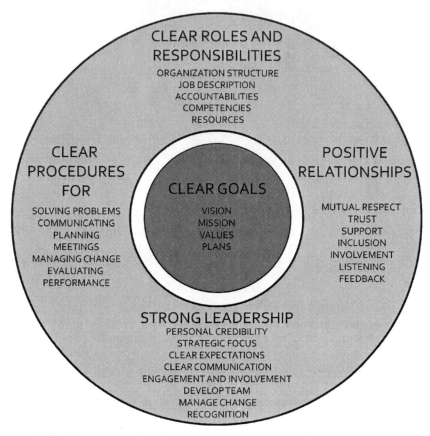

Figure 7.3: The University of Victoria team effectiveness model[3]

Understanding how to delegate and resolve conflict efficiently helps improve team dynamics and overall task performance.

Delegation

Delegation is the process of distributing responsibility for tasks to other members of an organisation or team. Advantages gained from delegation include the following.

➤ **Involvement** – Delegating tasks that carry significance give other members of the team a sense of personal involvement in projects. Subsequently, these members take ownership of the work being performed.
➤ **Motivation** – Involvement of team members and delegation of responsibility results in increased motivation.
➤ **Development** – Development of team member knowledge and skills arises from delegation of tasks.

➤ **Efficiency** – Delegation allows projects to be completed more efficiently, as members with appropriate knowledge and skills complete specific tasks.

Four main styles of delegation have been described.[4]

➤ **Controlling** – This style of delegation involves passing on tasks occasionally but strongly supervising. Consequently, individuals undertaking the task may feel they are not fully trusted and lack power.

➤ **Tentative** – These delegators will be more willing to delegate but will have several reservations. These may be related to doubts about the experience, capabilities and quality of work produced by others. They, therefore, take longer to pass on work and often only delegate parts of tasks. This reflects on the person undertaking the delegated tasks, who again may feel undervalued.

➤ **Participative** – In this style work is delegated to help individuals work in teams and experience differing tasks, which they may not have experienced before. This involves closely supervising individuals undertaking tasks.

➤ **Collaborative** – In this instance, individuals are selected to undertake tasks based on their expertise and background. In the early stages there is close working together to determine capabilities in performing the task. Later, they will collaborate as much or as little as is required.

Conflict

Conflict may be defined as any process caused by someone that may be perceived by someone else as negatively affecting something they care about. Conflict is often perceived as being a hindrance to progress; however, we will see that there are differing types of conflict, some of which are actually good for the organisation.

Types of conflict

➤ **Functional** – Some conflict may be productive and improve performance. This form of conflict, which is called functional or constructive conflict, may challenge existing processes and result in finding better alternatives hence improving outcomes.

➤ **Dysfunctional** – Dysfunctional or destructive conflict results in hindrance of performance.

➤ **Task** – Task conflict results when there are issues regarding the nature and goals of work.

➤ **Relationship** – This conflict arises from problems with interpersonal relationships.

➤ **Process** – Process conflict is related to how the work is undertaken.

Conflict process

The conflict process may be considered as a five-stage process (*see* Figure 7.4).[5]

Potential opposition or incompatibility

The first stage arises when there is a reason or condition that contributes to conflict potentially occurring. Three main broad conditions have been described as potential sources.

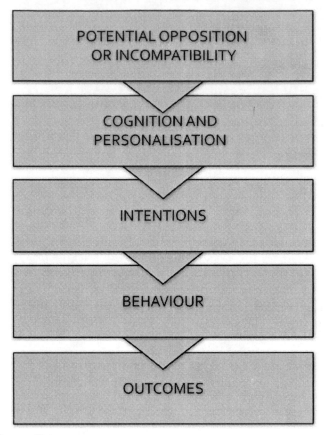

Figure 7.4: The conflict process

➤ **Communication** – Any problems in communication, such as use of medical terms, insufficient provision of information, language barriers, and can result in conflict.
➤ **Structure** – This refers to the size and specialisation of the team. Research shows that larger and more specialised teams tend to result in higher levels of conflict.
➤ **Personal variables** – Individuals will have their own values and characteristics which may not always be compatible with others thus giving rise to conflict.

Cognition and personalisation
In this stage, the reason for conflict becomes defined and both parties become aware that there is conflict. Personalisation occurs when the parties become emotionally involved, thus anxious, tense or hostile.

Intentions
Intentions are how the parties will react to the conflict. The perception by the other party of their intentions will influence how they will react. Thomas and Kilmann[6] identified a number of responses when faced with conflict. In these situations, an

individual's behaviour may be analysed according to assertiveness and cooperativeness. Assertiveness is the extent to which the individual attempts to satisfy their own concerns whilst cooperativeness attempts to satisfy the concerns of the other party. Based on the extent of these dimensions, the individual's conflict response can be defined as one of five modes (*see* Figure 7.5).

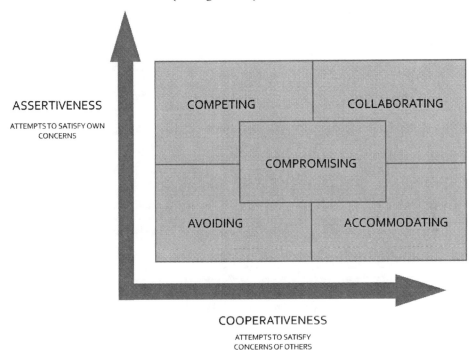

Figure 7.5: Thomas and Kilmann conflict responses[6]

➤ **Avoidance** – The individual pursues neither their concerns nor those of the other party. In doing so the individual avoids dealing with the conflict either by postponing or withdrawing from the situation.
➤ **Accommodation** – The individual aims to satisfy the concerns of the other individual and neglects their own concerns.
➤ **Competition** – Competing involves pursuing their own concerns and ignoring those of others. The aim is to win the conflict.
➤ **Compromise** – The aim is to find a mutually acceptable common ground where both parties concerns are partly met.
➤ **Collaboration** – This involves working together to find a solution that fully satisfies both concerns. The process requires in-depth discussion and analysis of the situation and exploring methods to come to a mutually beneficial solution. In this scenario, both parties win.
➤ **Behaviour** – This stage is how the individuals express their reaction to the conflict, whether verbal or even physical. This is a dynamic process with a rally of comments and actions between the players involved. The use of conflict resolution and stimulation techniques are employed to either de-escalate dysfunctional or escalate functional conflict (*see* Table 7.2).[7]

Table 7.2: Conflict management techniques[7]

Conflict resolution	
Problem solving	Identify and resolve with open communication.
Superordinate goals	Create shared goals that require cooperation from both parties.
Expansion of resources	If conflict arises from lack of resources then provision of further resources results in a solution.
Avoidance	Withdrawal or suppression.
Smoothing	Play down differences and emphasise common interests.
Compromise	Each party gives up something of value.
Authoritative command	Formal authority is used to determine the outcome.
Altering the human variable	Using behavioural change techniques.
Altering the structural variables	Changing the organisational structure.
Conflict stimulation	
Communication	Use of ambiguous or threatening messages to escalate conflict.
Bringing in outsiders	Employing people whose characteristics and values differ.
Restructuring the organisation	Changes in the organisational structure.
Appointing a devil's advocate	Purposely arguing against the team.

➤ **Outcomes** – The outcome of conflict may be functional or dysfunctional. Ideally, functional conflict should be encouraged to result in stimulated interaction between team members, sharing of ideas, creativity and better decision making.

Why the clinical team?

It is has become more and more apparent the medicine cannot be delivered by individuals without other allied professionals. The breadth and depth of medicine has reached such a stage that for optimum care patients will require the skills of numerous doctors and healthcare professionals.

The only way of effectively achieving this is the development of teams to deliver these healthcare processes. Every healthcare professional needs to understand that the team is important and doctors need to take leadership roles in this if it is going to be relevant to the practice of medicine.

The manger's role is to help all these direct front-line processes function in the most cost-effective ways. They should provide the systems, processes and structures to enable the whole process to work smoothly for the benefit of the patient. This has become more so in recent times with the complex financing of healthcare and greater accountability. Doctors and nurses need to take more of an advisory role in management. High performing clinical teams must not be disbanded to take up senior management as they do best in the clinical environment.

Working examples of a clinical team

In the outpatient clinical setting there is dynamic team that follows a patient pathway – the team forms and dissolves with each patient encounter. That functional SCU is very much a team although temporary but all the stages of the team formation has already occurred on a more permanent basis with the development of the outpatient team. Remember, you cannot work in isolation as a doctor – you may provide the best consultation but the patient experience can be poor due to a poor receptionist or nursing process or vice versa. Various targeted quality measurements tools can be used to measure these various members of the team.

Complex team processes with diverse skill sets are seen in the delivery of complex surgical procedures. Once again it may be temporary but the smooth and efficient dynamics of the team are essential to the delivery of safe and quality surgical outcomes. In critical incident analysis the team dynamics are an important part of the learning process for the team and healthcare organisation.

Multidisciplinary teams are an important part of the delivery of cancer care and the dynamics of the team are clearly seen here. They are a little more lasting and provide interprofessional and interspeciality contributions in the delivery of care for individual patients. These teams allow for measurement of team performance with specialised tools and are an excellent example of the clinical team at work.

Summary

The healthcare environment comprises a multitude of teams with varying functions. Functioning in teams is important in the effective and efficient delivery of quality healthcare. Understanding the anatomy and physiology of how teams are composed and function is essential in ensuring effectiveness and efficiency. This module has covered the conception and development of a team to managing the interactions within it.

Exercises

1   Consider the team you are currently part of and think of the individuals in that team. Classify each of those team members according to Belbin's team roles based on their strengths and weaknesses. Consider whether the individual roles compliment or hinder team progress.
2   Identify a goal which are you are aiming to achieve within a team. Use the team effectiveness model to define areas for improvement to help achieve this goal.
3   Think of a recent conflict scenario you have been involved in. Can you identify the different stages involved in the conflict? What was the outcome of the conflict? Could you now think of a collaborative solution, which would have been beneficial to both parties involved?

References

1   Tuckman BW. Developmental sequence in small groups. *Psychological Bulletin.* 1965; 63: 384–99.
2   Belbin RM. *Management Teams: why they succeed or fail.* Oxford: Butterworth Heinemann; 2002.
3   University of Victoria. *Team Effectiveness Model.* Available at: http://web.uvic.ca/hr/hrhandbook/organizdev/teammodel.pdf (accessed 31 May 2010).
4   Warner J. *Delegation.* Alresford: Management Pocketbooks; 2008.
5   Robbins SP. *Organisational Behaviour.* 10th ed. Upper Saddle River, NJ: Prentice Hall; 2003.
6   Thomas K, Kilmann R. *Thomas-Kilmann Conflict Mode Instrument.* Tuxedo, NY: Xicom Inc.; 1974.
7   Robbins SP. *Managing Organisational Conflict: a nontraditional approach.* Upper Saddle River, NJ: Prentice Hall; 1974.

Further reading

➤ West MA. *Effective Teamwork.* Oxford: Blackwell Publishing; 2004.
➤ West MA, Markiewicz L. *Building Team-Based Working.* Oxford: Blackwell Publishing; 2004.

Useful websites

Belbin: www.belbin.com/rte.asp?id=204

Clinical leaders

There are many definitions of leadership in the literature. Leadership has been defined in terms of traits, behaviour, influence, interactions, relationships and situations. However, a consistency in the definition revolves around the notion of a process whereby intentional influence is exerted by one person over other people to guide, structure and facilitate activities and relationships in a group or organisation.[1]

Study of leadership

Three major variables have been identified that are relevant in the understanding of leadership effectiveness (*see* Figure 8.1). These variables include characteristics of the:

➤ leader
➤ followers
➤ situation.

Most theories and empirical research exploring leadership may be classified into one of five approaches:

➤ trait
➤ behaviour
➤ power-influence
➤ situational
➤ integrative approach.

Trait approach

In 1869, Galton defined leadership as a unique property of extraordinary individuals whose decisions are capable of radically changing the streams of history, and that the unique attributes of such individuals is in their inherited makeup.[2] This led to interest in defining such personal qualities and the development of the trait theory of leadership.[3] During the 1930s and 1940s much research was conducted to elucidate these traits. However, in the late 1940s and 1950s, some reviews discarded the trait-based approaches of leadership as being insufficient to explain leadership and leader effectiveness.[4,5] Stodgill[4] concluded that:

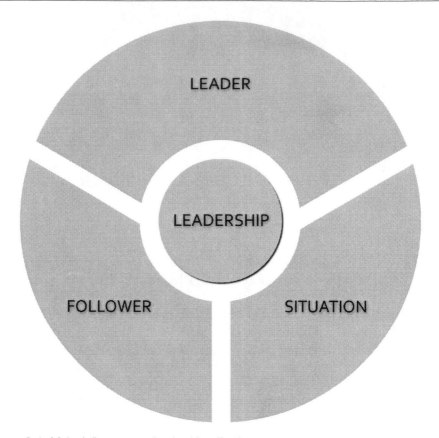

Figure 8.1: Major influences on leadership effectiveness

A person does not become a leader by virtue of the possession of some combination of traits ... the pattern of personal characteristics of the leader must bear some relevant relationship to the characteristics, activities, and goals of the followers.

There was a period of dormancy in the trait-based theory following this and it was not until the 1980s that a resurgence of research emerged challenging the rejection of trait-based theory.[5]

Behaviour approach

The behaviour approach began in the early 1950s when researchers were discouraged by the results of the trait-based approach. This approach investigated the role of the leader. The basis of this approach stemmed from two research studies performed by Ohio State University and the University of Michigan. The Ohio State study identified two broad categories of behaviour: consideration and initiating structure. Consideration was the concern of the leader for subordinates and their interpersonal relationships. Initiating structure was the leader concern for accomplishing the task.

The University of Michigan study identified three types of leadership behaviour: task-orientated behaviour; relations-orientated behaviour; and participative leadership. Results suggested that effective managers planned, organised and coordinated subordinates rather than doing the same kind of work as them. Effective managers were also more supportive and helpful to subordinates. Effective managers also used more group supervision instead of supervising individual subordinates.[1]

Power-influence approach

Power is the capacity to influence the attitudes and behaviour of people in the desired direction. Research into the power-influence approach examines the influence processes between leaders and other people. This research seeks to explain effectiveness in terms of the amount and type of power possessed by the leader and how it is exercised. There are a number of different types of power: reward; coercive; legitimate; expert; and referent. Research suggests that effective leaders rely more on personal power rather than positional power.

Situational approach

This approach, also known as contingency theory, emphasises the importance of contextual factors that influence the leadership process. The major situational variables include: characteristics of followers; nature of work; type of organisation; nature of external environment.

Integrative approach

An integrative approach involves more than one type of leadership variable. Recently, researchers have been adopting the use of different theories within the same studies. An example of the integrative approach would be transactional and transformational leadership.

Transactional and transformational leadership

In 1978, Burns introduced the distinction between transactional and transformational leaders.[6] Transformational leaders offer a purpose that transcends short-term goals and focuses on higher order intrinsic needs. Transactional leaders, in contrast, focus on proper exchange of resources.[7] Burns described transactional and transformational leadership representing opposite ends of a single continuum (*see* Figure 8.2).[6]

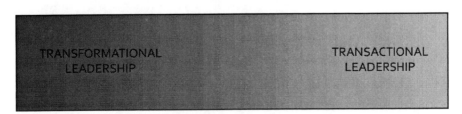

Figure 8.2: Burns' model of transactional and transformational leadership[6]

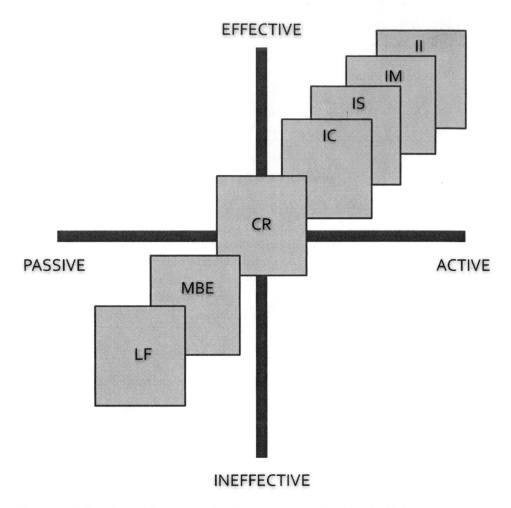

Figure 8.3: Bass's model of transactional and transformational leadership[8]

In 1985, Bass, basing his work on the concepts raised by Burns, developed several modifications.[8] He postulated that transactional and transformational leadership were separate concepts and that leaders could be both transactional and transformational (*see* Figure 8.3). He has shown that some of the best leaders exhibited both transactional and transformational styles.[9]

Bass elaborated the original concept further and identified eight dimensions of leadership behaviour.[8] The four dimensions of transformational leadership are as follows.

➤ **Idealised influence** refers to leaders who have high standards of moral and ethical conduct, who are held in high personal regard, and who engender loyalty from followers.
➤ **Inspirational motivation** is the degree to which the leader articulates a vision that is appealing and inspiring to followers. *Charisma*, often used to represent a combination of idealised influence and inspirational motivation, is the degree

to which the leader behaves in admirable ways that cause followers to identify with the leader.

➤ **Intellectual stimulation** is the degree to which the leader challenges assumptions, takes risks and solicits followers' ideas.
➤ **Individualised consideration** is the degree to which the leader attends to each follower's needs, acts as a mentor to the follower, and listens to the follower's concerns and needs.[10]

The three dimensions of transactional leadership are as follows.

➤ **Contingent reward** refers to leadership behaviours focused on exchange of resources.
➤ **Management by exception-active** refers to monitoring performance and taking corrective action as necessary. In contrast,
➤ **Management by exception-passive** leaders take a passive approach only intervening when problems become serious.[11]

The final leadership dimension is *laissez-faire*, which is the avoidance or absence of any leadership. Researchers have argued this final dimension should be treated separately from transformational and transactional leadership.[12]

Transformational leadership has become one of the dominant leadership theories. Research studies have found relationships between transformational leadership and followers' commitment, loyalty, satisfaction and performance.[13,14] Transformational leadership, in a medical context, has been positively associated with service quality and achievement of disease management goals.[15,16]

Becoming a transformational leader

We have seen that transformational leadership has been shown to have many positive influences on the working environment and performance. The question arises as to whether these leadership skills are inherently present in certain individuals or if they can be learned.

Case study

What is a leader? Are plastic surgeons leaders?

A web-based survey of consultant plastic surgeons was performed, assessing their leadership behaviour. This survey revealed that the 44 consultants who replied had moderate mean scores for transformational and transactional leadership behaviours. The mean score for *laissez-faire* behaviour was low. The study concluded that this group of plastic surgeons inherently exhibited moderate degrees of transformational and transactional behaviour. It has been suggested that increasing awareness of leadership behaviours and how to enhance them can improve leadership skills.

Certain individuals will be more charismatic and inspirational than others, but most skills of transformational leadership may be learned. So how can we develop the skills necessary to become a more transformational leader? Based on the four dimensions described above, we can begin to understand how transformational leaders exert their influence. Exploring these dimensions allows us to produce some guidance for becoming a more transformational leader. Below are some pointers to help develop these skills.

➤ **Develop a clear vision and effectively communicate this** – A clear vision must have a specific set target that is obtainable within a set time frame. For example, in our clinic we will reduce the rate of coronary heart disease deaths by 50% within the next year.

➤ **Do the right thing** – Make decision-making consistent and transparent to fellow team members. Consistency and application of the same rules to all allows followers to build trust and respect in their leader.

➤ **Motivate and show optimism** – Providing followers with inspiration and belief in their work helps motivate them to achieve more. The use of phrases such as 'I believe that you can do this' can prove to be highly motivating to individuals and give them a meaning of self-worth.

➤ **Empower team members** – Involve followers in decision-making and make them feel as though they are part of the team. Ask them 'What would you do or advise me?' This provides followers with a feeling of self-worth and control, and intellectually stimulates them.

➤ **Respond to the needs of individuals** – Be available to your followers and provide them with time to voice their needs. Provide support for individuals and mentor, coach or counsel them when required. Recognise good performance and acknowledge this.

These pointers provide a foundation for developing transformational leadership skills. To further these skills, leaders should seek development workshops and obtain feedback from their followers. Individualised consideration requires further development of skills necessary to provide mentoring and coaching.

Mentoring and coaching

There is often confusion about exactly what mentoring and coaching mean and some use these terms interchangeably. There is, however, a distinction between the two terms as we shall see below.

Mentoring

Mentoring is process whereby senior employees provide guidance and direction to less experienced members of the team. This tends to be a long-term relationship that explores not only performance at work but also personal and career develop-ment. The mentor–protégé relationship not only brings benefits to both parties concerned but also to the organisation in which they work. These benefits include the following.

Mentor benefits
➤ Personal satisfaction.
➤ Sharing of experience and knowledge.

➤ Enhanced and direct communication with employees.
➤ Source of alternative perspectives.
➤ Communication of organisational culture and roles.

Protégé benefits
➤ Improved skills and knowledge.
➤ Shortened learning curve of new roles.
➤ Increased motivation and empowerment.
➤ Enhanced career progression.
➤ Opportunities for networking.

Organisational benefits
➤ Higher employee satisfaction.
➤ Improved performance and delivery of services.
➤ Greater commitment to organisation and employee retention.
➤ Shows organisational commitment to growth of its employees.
➤ Enhanced communication within organisation.

Alred *et al.*[17] describe mentoring as a three-stage process (*see* Figure 8.4), which involves the following.

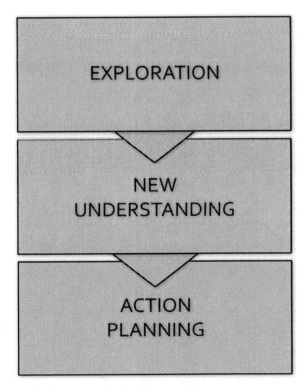

Figure 8.4: Three stages of the mentoring process[17]

➤ **Exploration** – The mentor negotiates an agenda by listening to the protégé. The aim and objectives of the mentoring are clarified by summarising the needs of the protégé. It is crucial that commitment is shown and a rapport is established with the protégé to encourage exploration.

➤ **New understanding** – This stage involves providing constructive feedback, support and counselling to the protégé. It also involves demonstration of skills and coaching. The mentor recognises the strengths and weaknesses and identifies the developmental needs. The process of giving information and advice is undertaken. Sharing one's own experiences and stories helps consolidate the protégé's learning during this stage.

➤ **Action planning** – This stage encourages new and creative ways of thinking. The mentor helps examine the options for action and their consequences. Finally, the protégé and mentor negotiate an action plan. Progress is monitored and evaluated to see if the outcomes laid out in the action plan have been achieved.

Coaching

A process whereby an individual, through direct discussion and guided activity, helps a colleague to learn to solve a problem, or to do a task, better than would otherwise be the case.[18] Coaching is a short-term relationship that focuses on improvement of performance in a specific task. This differs from mentoring, which tends to be a longer relationship exploring many aspects of the protégé's needs.

Coaching focuses on improving specific skills. Coaching in sport provides a process framework that relies on three main elements.

➤ **The game plan** – the tactics to win the game.
➤ **Watching the play** – monitoring performance.
➤ **Time out** – providing feedback.

The coaching process

➤ **Defining the goals** – The goals should be specific and skills focused. The coach and coachee should have a clear vision of the aim of the process.
➤ **Analysis of current practice** – Assessment of the current skill level of the coachee is made.
➤ **Exploration of options to achieve goals** – The greatest limitation to success lies with the self-belief of the individual regarding what can be achieved. The role of the coach is to identify such limiting thoughts, provide positive reinforcement and develop the self-confidence of the individual.
➤ **Implement agreed actions**.
➤ **Feedback** – This is an important part of the coaching process. Feedback should be open and honest. Feedback focus should revolve around future tactics that complement the strengths of the individual. When giving negative feedback, the focus should be on the process, result or tactic rather than personal qualities of the individual. An opportunity to correct the behaviour in question should be given soon after such feedback. This avoids the individuals dwelling on the criticisms and considering themselves as a failure.

Coaching may be used in clinical teams when training juniors to undertake specific tasks. Coaching has also been used in medicine to enhance patient care in chronic conditions. The coaching of patients in these situations is to identify the clinical and personal priorities in their care and agree on a management plan. Coaching has been shown to have a positive impact on patients' knowledge, information recall and participation in the decision-making process.[19]

Summary

The leader is an important part of any clinical team. Transformational leaders have been shown to produce more effective performance from their followers, who demonstrate loyalty and higher satisfaction. The methods used by transformational leaders can be learned and developed. A leader must also be an effective mentor and coach to their followers.

Exercises

1   Think of a leader whom you admire – this maybe someone at work or well-known figure. Consider the dimensions of transformational and transactional leadership behaviour and identify these dimensions in your chosen leader. Do you find that they tend to exhibit more transformational leadership behaviour? Consider what methods they use to motivate and inspire followers.
2   Consider a recent time when you have been a leader, whether at work, during sport or in any other situation. How did you lead the team? Did you achieve your goal? Did you feel that you inspired your team? Did the team feel involved? How could you have achieved your goal more efficiently and effectively?
3   Think of a situation where you have supervised a more junior colleague or tried to teach someone a task. How did you go about undertaking this? Can you identify steps you could have undertaken to help coach this individual more effectively?

References

1   Yukl GA. *Leadership in Organizations.* Upper Saddle River, NJ: Pearson Prentice Hall; 2006.
2   Galton F. *Hereditary Genius.* New York: Appleton; 1869.
3   Judge TA, Bono JE, Ilies R, *et al.* Personality and leadership: a qualitative and quantitative review. *Journal of Applied Psychology.* 2002; **87**: 765–80.
4   Stodgill RM. Personal factors associated with leadership: a survey of the literature. *Journal of Psychology.* 1948; **25**: 35–71.
5   Zaccaro SJ. Trait-based perspectives of leadership. *American Psychologist.* 2007; **62**: 6–16.
6   Burns JM. *Leadership.* New York: Harper and Row; 1978.
7   Conger JA, Kanungo RN. *Charismatic Leadership in Organizations.* Thousand Oaks, CA: Sage; 1998.
8   Bass BM. *Leadership and Performance Beyond Expectations.* New York: Free Press; 1985.

9 Bass BM. Two decades of research and development in transformational leadership. *European Journal of Work and Organizational Psychology.* 1999; **8**: 9–32.

10 Judge TA, Piccolo RF. Transformational and transactional leadership: a meta-analytic test of their relative validity. *Journal of Applied Psychology.* 2004; **89**: 755–68.

11 Bono JE, Judge TA. Personality and transformational and transactional leadership: a meta-analysis. *Journal of Applied Psychology.* 2004; **89**: 901–10.

12 Bass BM, Riggio RE. *Transformational Leadership.* 2nd ed. Mahwah, NJ: Lawrence Erlbaum Associates; 2006.

13 Lim B, Polyhart RE. Transformational leadership: relations to the five-factor model and team performance in typical and maximum contexts. *Journal of Applied Psychology.* 2004; **89**: 610–21.

14 Niehoff BP, Enz CA, Grover RA. The impact of top-management actions on employees' attitudes. *Group and Organizational Management.* 1995; **15**: 337–52.

15 Jabnoun N, Al Rasasi AJ. Transformational leadership and service quality in UAE hospitals. *Managing Service Quality.* 2005; **15**: 70–81.

16 Xirasagar S, Samuels PH, Curtin TF. Management training of physician executives, their leadership style, and care management performance: an empirical study. *American Journal of Managed Care.* 2006; **12**: 101–8.

17 Alred G, Garvey B, Smith R. *The Mentoring Pocketbook.* Alresford: Management Pocketbooks Ltd; 1998.

18 Megginson D, Boydell T. *A Manager's Guide to Coaching.* London: CIPD; 1979.

19 Coutler A, Ellins J. Effectiveness of strategies for informing, educating and involving patients. *British Medical Journal.* 2007; **335**: 24–7.

Case studies

Nassab R. What is a leader? Are plastic surgeons leaders? *Plastic and Reconstructive Surgery.* 2010; **125**: 1049–50.

Further reading

➤ Hughes RL, Ginnett RC, Curphy GJ. *Leadership.* Boston: Irwin McGraw Hill; 1996.

➤ Yukl GA. *Leadership in Organizations.* Upper Saddle River, NJ: Pearson Prentice Hall; 2006.

Useful websites

NHS Leadership Qualities Framework: www.nhsleadershipqualities.nhs.uk/

NHS Institute for Innovation and Improvement: www.institute.nhs.uk/building_capability/general/leadership_home.html

Chartered Institute of Personnel and Development – Leadership: www.cipd.co.uk/subjects/maneco/leadership/leadshipovw.htm

Managing clinicians' performance

Defining performance

Paraphrasing from Max Moullin's one recommendation of defining performance:[1] clinical performance of a doctor is how well they manage the patient pathway and the value they deliver to the patient, the clinical team, and the community in utilising their resources efficiently and effectively.

It is important for any system of measuring doctor performance to be credible. Quality assurance of medical practice and professional self-regulation must incorporate elements of outcome assessment and peer review.[2]

What do we measure?

We need to measure the doctor's role in managing his patient's pathway, which is the complete clinical episode. This has to be unique to the doctor's practice and generic performance indicators are not useful for the clinician. So the doctor has to take ownership and work with the management team in developing what needs to be measured. The required standard to be compared against needs to be identified for that particular process. Index clinical processes are determined for that particular doctor's practice and agreed upon. This baseline standard is also agreed and the doctor's performance is then measured against it.

The public want all doctors to recognise the following.[3]

➤ Good communication is essential in the medical consultation.
➤ When they so choose, patients wish to make up their own minds about their options for the management of their illness.
➤ Patronising or arrogant behaviour is unacceptable.
➤ The profession should show its determination to confront poor practice and end the secrecy that surrounds it.
➤ Doctors should be prepared to accept more accountability, individually and collectively.
➤ The profession should be tough on serious misconduct, such as sexual misconduct with patients or disregard for patients' safety in clinical practice.

➤ The public's insistence that their expectations be addressed, and the growing recognition within the profession that they must be, are leading to change in the culture of doctors' professionalism.

Irvine's paper[3] was the initiator for the development of the Good Medical Practice of the General Medical Council in the UK. The American Medical Association (AMA)-convened Physician Consortium for Performance Improvement (PCPI) aims to enhance quality of care and patient safety through development, testing, and maintenance of evidence-based clinical performance measures and measurement resources for physicians.[4]

Patient pathway

Using the patient pathway for a surgical episode (*see* Figure 9.1), we can measure performance for each domain on the pathway with different tools. For example at the consultation point, the SERVQUAL tool can be used to measure the quality of the consultation using the areas of reliability, assurance, tangible, empathy and

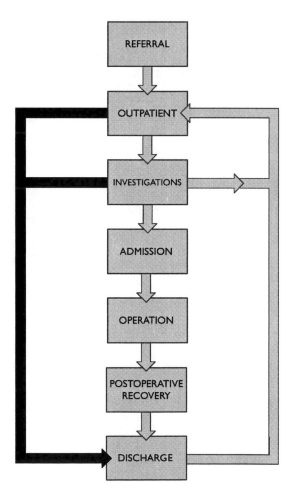

Figure 9.1: Surgical pathway

responsiveness. The SERVQUAL tool is discussed further in the operations module. The questionnaires have to be carefully designed, administered and analysed regularly for them to be effective. For adequate preoperative assessment, the cancellation rate due to inadequate preoperative workup will indicate a good measure. Surgical theatre utilisation shows effective resource use by the doctor and the average surgical time for standard procedures shows performance issues clearly. Complication rates are used universally in audits but their effectiveness has not been conclusively proven to affect performance.

Key performance indicators (KPI) for clinicians

Once we have determined what needs to be measured, we then need to develop the KPI for a doctor. These are quantifiable measurements, agreed beforehand by the doctor and the management, that reflect the critical success factors of the healthcare organisation. The doctor must be engaged in this exercise to help management identify what are the specific KPI for him and the role of management is to help gather the data so that the doctor can assess his performance. The whole principle of performance management is to help the doctor outperform himself. The purpose of this process is reflective learning, self and continuous improvement. KPIs are playing a key role in changing the locus of performance assessment along two dimensions: location and expertise.[5]

These KPIs then need to be included in the annual appraisal documents of the individual doctor. In the UK, all consultant doctors have to undergo an annual appraisal process taking into account all the domains that are required as a professional with good practice. The appraisal is about helping individuals to improve the way they work and the services they provide.

In the United States, the AMA's PCPI currently has over 260 performance measures covering many aspect of healthcare, an example of which is given below.[4]

AMA's PCPI Measures for Melanoma

Measure 1 – Follow-up aspects of care.
Percentage of patients, regardless of age, with a new diagnosis of melanoma or a history of melanoma who received all of the following aspects of care within the 12 month reporting period: (1) Patient was asked about new and changing moles **AND** (2) Patient received a complete physical skin examination **AND** (3) Patient was counseled to perform a monthly self skin examination.

Measure 2 – Continuity of care – recall system.
Percentage of patients, regardless of age, with a current diagnosis of melanoma or a history of melanoma whose information was entered, at least once within a 12 month period into a recall system that includes:
- A target date for the next complete physical skin exam, AND
- A process to follow up with patients who either did not make an appointment within the specified timeframe or who missed a scheduled appointment

Measure 3 – Coordination of care.
Percentage of patient visits, regardless of age, seen with a new occurrence of melanoma who have a treatment plan documented in the chart that was communicated to the physician(s) providing continuing care within one month of diagnosis.

Measure 4 – Appropriate use of imaging studies in stage 0–1A melanoma.
Percentage of patients, regardless of age, with Stage 0 or 1A melanoma, without signs or symptoms, for whom no diagnostic imaging studies have been ordered related to the melanoma diagnosis.

What matters most?

At the end of the day we want to measure the performance of doctors so that patients get the best care in the most cost-effective manner and with minimal risk to patients. Any performance management system has to take into account patient outcomes. At the same time doctors must realise that resources are not unlimited and must understand the cost of care.

Why manage performance?

The assessment of work performance is considered central to definitions of professional autonomy.[4] As part of the reflective practice of all doctors, they will need to measure their performance. These measures need to be specific. The public and healthcare providers and legislation now require performance management as part of the accreditation and credentialing process for the doctor in most countries.

The earliest strategies, which included continuing professional education, clinical audits, and peer review, were aimed at the individual doctor, and produced only modest effects. Other efforts, such as national implementation of practice guidelines, effective use of information technologies, and intensive involvement by doctors in continuous quality-improvement activities, are aimed more broadly at healthcare systems.[6]

The UK government and doctors' groups have agreed to an ambitious incentive scheme to be implemented through primary care trusts, in which family doctors will be paid against performance assessed on 76 quality indicators in 10 clinical domains of care, 56 indicators in organisational areas and four indicators relating to patients' experience. Implementation of this bold proposal will be challenging. Here we see the regulators and funders are putting money behind their collective objectives to incentivise doctors to obtain desirable patient outcomes.

Who drives performance?

There are a number of drivers for performance (*see* Figure 9.2), these involve the following.

Doctor

For any performance management system to be effective it has to have ownership of the group to be managed. As doctors are crucial to the delivery of care they have to be actively engaged and involved in developing and implementing the performance management system. It has to be a bottom-up approach with the guidelines given and the doctors allowed to develop it from the bottom up. The grass root doctors know what they are doing and what parameters need to be measured. The role of management is to enable this whole process and there must be sufficient allocation

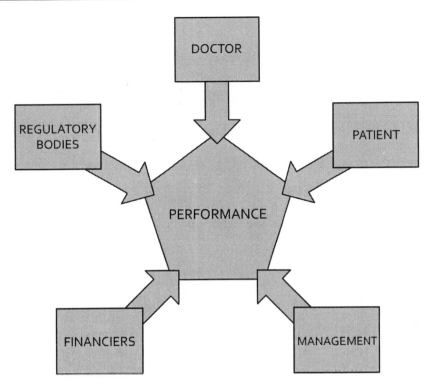

Figure 9.2: Drivers of performance

of resources for this to happen. It also becomes easier to manage underperformers, as it was the doctors who developed the system and set the criteria. The management role is just to facilitate the measurement and make such data available for the doctors.

Patients

As the consumers of healthcare, the patients are key in driving quality and therefore performance of doctors. They play an important role in providing feedback in managing the performance of the doctors. The whole purpose of the doctor's role is to serve their patients. This can be achieved with the use of 360-degree feedback or multi-source feedback (MSF) is being developed whose purpose is to provide a sample of attitudes and opinions of colleagues and patients on the work performance of the person concerned. This tool measures a doctor figuratively in the centre of the circle of the clinical environment. Subordinates, peers and supervisors provide feedback. It also includes a self-assessment and, in some cases, feedback from external sources such as non-clinical staff like secretaries and clerks, and can include medical suppliers or other interested stakeholders. Patient questionnaires to measure doctor performance can be misleading if poorly designed.

The Picker Institute,[7] in an independent healthcare experts study, reviewed a selection of questionnaires currently being used to gather feedback from patients on individual doctors, including those used by GPs to gain additional contract points under the Quality and Outcomes Framework, and it makes a number of key recommendations.

> The development of questionnaires that focus more on patient engagement and include a fuller range of questions.
> Further research on what topics it is appropriate to ask patients to provide feedback on, including aspects of a doctor's technical competence.
> The development of questionnaires that tackle specific conditions or specialties.
> Closer examination of the best ways to administer feedback surveys in clinical settings.

There are various other tools available for measuring the patient expectation and perception of quality of care delivered.[8]

Regulatory bodies

In the UK, the General Medical Council (GMC)[9] introduced the licence to practise in 2009:

> *... to practise medicine in the UK all doctors are required by law to hold both registration and a licence to practise. This applies whether they practise full time, part time, as a locum, privately or in the NHS, or whether they are employed or self-employed. Licensing is the first practical step towards the introduction of a new system called revalidation. This will require doctors to renew their licence to practise periodically. The purpose of revalidation will be to give patients regular assurance that doctors registered with a licence are up to date and fit to practise.*

For revalidation, the GMC states three elements:

> To confirm that licensed doctors practise in accordance with the GMC's generic standards.
> To confirm that doctors on the GMC's specialist register or GP register continue to meet the standards appropriate for their specialty.
> To identify for further investigation, and remediation, poor practice where local systems are not robust enough to do this or do not exist.

Financiers of healthcare

In the fee for service environment and also more now in the public sector, doctors have to be accountable for the cost of delivering their care. It is no longer acceptable that doctors can perform clinical processes for their patient without taking cost into consideration. It is the responsibility of the doctor to weigh all the factors in deciding on a management strategy that will be most cost-effective and beneficial to the patient.

Haslam found that additional hospital funding has not delivered robust financials in the four nation's hospital sector and that physical transformation is limited and fragile. So more money does not necessarily mean better outcomes.[10] There is evidence showing the role of incentives is not only to motivate high performance through the alignment of results and rewards (financial/non-financial as well as direct/indirect) but also to enable healthcare providers to perform better by mitigating financial barriers that typically result from funding schemes.[11]

Management

Jacobs *et al.* found that although there was some interest in cost and activity information among doctors, clinical staff generally did not have access to it.[12] Cost and activity information was only available to clinical staff at the most senior levels. Therefore, serious questions must be raised about the extent of penetration that these reforms have had at the clinical level. It is the management's role to ensure that the information is made available to the front-liners to ensure high performance.

Managers have a significant role to play in the performance of their doctors. They need to provide the resources necessary for the doctors to perform and also help them measure their performance so that the mangers can fulfil their role in cost-effective quality healthcare delivery.

Rodger *et al.* found that a significant relationship was observed between the management of healthcare information and quality performance. IT infrastructure exhibited a direct, rather than a moderating, effect on quality performance. The research also found that significant differences exist between customer and manager perceptions of quality.[13]

How to manage doctors' performance

According to the Department of Health UK,[14] the appraisal:

> ... *offers a framework for planned, constructive, professional dialogue. It provides the opportunity for reflection about current performance and progress. This is used as a platform to set goals for future professional practice and development which will also contribute to the needs of the organisation in which the individual works. Appraisal should therefore be a positive, constructive process which is mutually beneficial to both the individuals being appraised and also to the organisation in which they work.*

Good Medical Practice sets out the principles and values on which good practice are founded; these principles together describe medical professionalism in action. The guidance is addressed to doctors, but it is also intended to let the public know what they can expect from doctors.

The domains to be measured in the doctors' appraisal include (taken from the GMC):[15]

1. GOOD MEDICAL PRACTICE

A. GOOD MEDICAL CARE
Examples of documentation which may be appropriate:

- Current job plan/work programme.
- Indicative information regarding annual caseload/workload.
- Up-to-date audit data including information on audit methodology if available.
- Record of how results of audit have resulted in changes to practice (if applicable).
- Results of clinical outcomes as compared to relevant royal college, faculty or specialty association recommendations where available.
- Evidence of any resource shortfalls which may have compromised outcomes.
- Evidence of how any in-service educational activity may have affected service delivery.
- Records of outcome of any investigated formal complaints in which the investigation has been completed in the past 12 months, or since doctors last appraisal.
- A description of how the outcome of any complaints has resulted in changes to practice.
- Outcome of external reviews (peer and otherwise).
- A description of any issues arising in relation to adherence to employer clinical governance policies.
- Record of how relevant clinical guidelines are reviewed by the appraisee and his/her team and how these have affected practice.
- Records of any relevant critical incident reports.
- Any other routine indicators of the standards of the doctors care which the doctor uses.

B. MAINTAINING GOOD MEDICAL PRACTICE

The purpose of this section is to record continuous professional development CPD/CME activities undertaken since the last appraisal. Any difficulties in attending CPD/CME activities should be recorded, with reasons.

Examples of documentation which may be appropriate (if available):

- Examples of participation in appropriate Continuing Professional Development, this might include individual development activity, locally-based development and participation in college or specialty association activities.
- List all CPD courses attended, and points awarded for each attendance.

C. WORKING RELATIONSHIPS WITH COLLEAGUES

The purpose of this section is to reflect on doctors relationships with doctors colleagues.

Examples of documentation which may be appropriate:

- A description of the setting within which you work and the team structure within which you practise.
- Any other documentary evidence that may be available (such as records of any formal peer reviews or discussions) should be included here, otherwise a record of the discussion and any action agreed should form part of the summary.

D. RELATIONS WITH PATIENTS

The purpose of this section is to reflect the doctors' relationships with his patients.

Examples of documentation which may be appropriate:

- Any examples of good practice or concern in doctors relationships with patients
- A description of doctors approach to handling informed consent.
- This might include validated patients surveys, doctors assessment of any changes in doctors practice as a result of any investigated complaint, compliments from patients, peer reviews/surveys.

E. TEACHING AND TRAINING

The purpose of this section is to reflect on doctors teaching and training activities since doctors last appraisal. Any difficulties in arranging cover for doctors clinical work whilst undertaking teaching and training (including educational activities for the NHS generally) should be recorded.

Examples of documentation which may be appropriate:

- A summary of formal teaching/lecturing activities, supervision/mentoring duties, any recorded feedback from those taught.

F. PROBITY

The doctor should note here any concerns raised or problems encountered during the year on either of these issues and include any records.

G. HEALTH

The doctor should note here any concerns raised or problems encountered during the year on either of these issues and include any records.

2. MANAGEMENT ACTIVITY

Examples of documentation which may be appropriate:

* Information about doctors formal management commitments, records of any noteworthy achievements and any recorded feedback if available.

This section provides an opportunity to add any further information, including any difficulties in arranging cover for doctors' clinical work whilst undertaking management activity including activities for the NHS regionally and nationally.

3. RESEARCH

Examples of documentation which may be appropriate:

* Evidence of formal research commitments.
* Record of any research ongoing or completed in the previous year.
* Record of funding arrangements for research.
* Record of noteworthy achievements.
* Confirmation that appropriate ethical approval has been secured for all research undertaken.

4. REPORT ON DEVELOPMENT ACTION IN THE PAST YEAR

The doctor should summarise here the development action agreed at the last appraisal (or at any interim meeting) or include doctor's personal development plan. This will facilitate discussion on progress towards development goals. You should record where it is agreed that goals have been achieved or where further action is required. It is assumed that where a development need has not been met in full it will remain a need and will either be reflected in the coming year's plan or have resulted in other action.

Summary

Measuring performance of clinicians is important. There are many drivers for performance in a clinical setting including the doctor, patient, regulatory bodies, stakeholders, and management. Measuring performance allows further improvement in the provision of care in an effective and efficient manner. Performance measurement is now also part of the appraisal process for doctors and subsequently essential for licensing to practice medicine. The GMC has provided guidance on domains for assessment of clinician's performance.

Exercises

1   Consider your daily work and the activities you undertake. Can you identify how you could objectively measure your performance? Are there any guidelines for the KPI you have identified? Are you achieving these targets?

2   Consider each of these KPI. What are the targets that are set? Who has drawn up these targets? What are the benefits to you, the patient and management of these targets?

3   Using the AMA's PCPI measures available on the AMA website, consider a condition relevant to your practice. Assess your performance based on the PCPI measures.

4   Using the GMC guidance on Good Medical Practice, identify and record activities for each dimension. This provides evidence for your forthcoming annual appraisal. Are there any areas of concern that require improvement?

References

1   Moullin M. Defining performance measurement. *Perspectives on Performance.* 2003; 2(2): 3.

2   Lim TO, Soraya A, Ding LM, *et al.* Assessing doctors' competence: application of CUSUM technique in monitoring doctors' performance. *International Journal of Quality in Health Care.* 2002; 14(3): 251–8.

3   Irvine D. The performance of doctors: the new professionalism. *The Lancet.* 1999; 353(9159): 1174–7.

4   American Medical Association. *Physician Consortium for Performance Improvement.* Available at: www.ama-assn.org/ama/pub/physician-resources/clinical-practice-improvement/clinical-quality/physician-consortium-performance-improvement.shtml (accessed 31 May 2010).

5   Exworthy M, Wilkinson EK, McColl A, *et al.* The role of performance indicators in changing the autonomy of the general practice profession in the UK. *Social Science and Medicine.* 2003; 56(7): 1493–504.

6   Lanier DC, Roland M, Burstin H, *et al.* Doctor performance and public accountability. *The Lancet.* 2003; 362: 1404–8.

7   Chisholm A, Askham J. *What Do You Think of Your Doctor?* Oxford: Picker Institute Europe; 2006.

8   Lee H, Delene LM, Bunda MA, *et al.* Methods of measuring health-care service quality. *Journal of Business Research.* 2000; 48(3): 233–46.

9   General Medical Council. *Registration and Licensing.* Available at: www.gmc-uk.org/doctors/index.asp (accessed 31 May 2010).

10 Haslam C, Marriott N. Accounting for reform: funding and transformation in the four nation's hospital services. *Accounting Forum.* 2006; 30(4): 389–405.

11 Custers T, Klazinga NS, Brown AD. Increasing performance of health care services within economic constraints: working towards improved incentive structures. *German Journal for Quality in Health Care.* 2007; 101(6): 381–8.

12 Jacobs K, Marcon G, Witt D. Cost and performance information for doctors: an international comparison. *Management Accounting Research.* 2004; 15(3): 337–54.

13 Rodger JA, Pendharkar PC, Paper DJ. Management of information technology and quality performance in health care facilities. *International Journal of Applied Quality Management.* 1999; 2(2): 251–69.

14 Department of Health. *Appraisals.* Available at: http://webarchive.nationalarchives. gov.uk/+/www.dh.gov.uk/en/Managingyourorganisation/Workforce/Education-TrainingandDevelopment/Appraisals/index.htm (accessed 31 May 2010).

15 General Medical Council. *Good Medical Practice.* Available at: www.gmc-uk.org/ static/documents/content/GMC_GMP_0911.pdf (accessed 31 May 2010).

Case example

American Medical Association. *Physician Consortium for Performance Improvement – Measures for Melanoma.* Available at: www.ama-assn.org/ama1/pub/upload/mm/370/ melanoma-worksheets.pdf (accessed 31 May 2010).

Useful websites

American Medical Association – Code of Medical Ethics: www.ama-assn.org/ama/pub/ physician-resources/medical-ethics/code-medical-ethics.shtml

American Medical Association – Physician Consortium for Performance Improvement: www.ama-assn.org/ama/pub/physician-resources/clinical-practice-improvement/ clinical-quality/physician-consortium-performance-improvement.shtml

General Medical Council: www.gmc-uk.org

NHS Institute for Innovation and Improvement – Performance Management: www. institute.nhs.uk/quality_and_service_improvement_tools/quality_and_service_ improvement_tools/performance_management.html

The learning and teaching clinician

Clinicians spend a significant portion of their time learning and developing their knowledge and skills. Many clinicians also become teachers, both in a formal or informal environment. This module explores how individuals learn and provides guidance on how to plan a learning event.

Learning

Many theories relating to learning have been described, varying from conditioning (Pavlov's dogs) to more recent e-learning concepts. One of the most frequently used theories was popularised by Kolb. Kolb described learning as the process whereby knowledge is created through the transformation of experience.[1]

Experiential learning model

In 1976, Kolb proposed the experiential learning model, which describes how people learn.[2] This theory emphasises the crucial role of experience in the learning process. This model has become more commonly known as the Kolb Learning Cycle (*see* Figure 10.1).

It consists of four main stages, which describe how experience is translated into concepts that are then used as guides in the choice of new experiences. The stages are as follows.

➤ **Concrete experience** – The learner must become fully and openly immersed, without bias, in the new experience. This stage involves learning from specific experiences or other people's experiences.
➤ **Reflective observation** – This stage is the reflection and observation of experiences from different perspectives, which involves looking back at what and how things were done.
➤ **Abstract conceptualisation** – This is the process of creating concepts that integrate the reflections and observations with previous or new knowledge into sound theories.
➤ **Active experimentation** – Active experimentation involves the application of the new theories to solve problems and make decisions. This stage involves doing the task at hand.

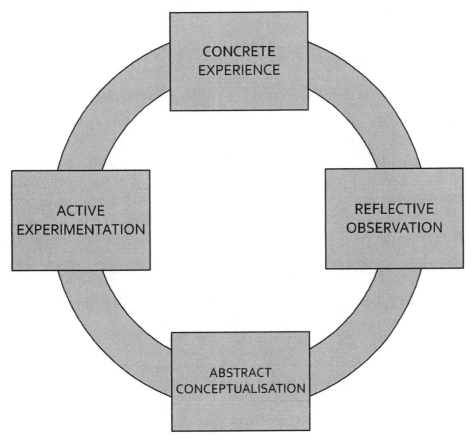

Figure 10.1: Kolb learning cycle[2]

The cycle may be entered at any stage depending on the circumstances and situation. Once the cycle has been entered the subsequent steps are taken in order to learn.

Example

An intern or junior doctor would like to learn to perform central venous cannulation.

Reflective observation – Junior has been thinking about task and seen senior undertake it.
Abstract conceptualisation – Understanding the theory and anatomy relating to the technique.
Active experimentation – Performing the task.
Concrete experience – Receiving tips from colleagues.

Types of learner

In 1992, Honey and Mumford described four learning styles, each of which is strongly associated with the stages of the learning cycle (*see* Figure 10.2).[3] These learning styles are as follows.

➤ **Activists** – These individuals thrive on challenges posed by new experience and will try anything once. They are not interested in long-term consolidation and prefer short-term crisis.
➤ **Reflectors** – Reflectors tend to step back and reflect on the experience from different perspectives. They are cautious and will gather all the information, and consider the possible options before making a decision.
➤ **Theorists** – Theorists or analysts are systematic logical thinkers who like theories and models. Theorists often dislike creative or subjective thinking.
➤ **Pragmatists** – Pragmatists respond to problems and opportunities as challenges. They seek out new ideas and theories that may be applicable to their situation, and experiment with them.

The Kolb learning cycle and the above learning types are frequently used in adult learning theory. They form a useful foundation to further understanding of the learning process.

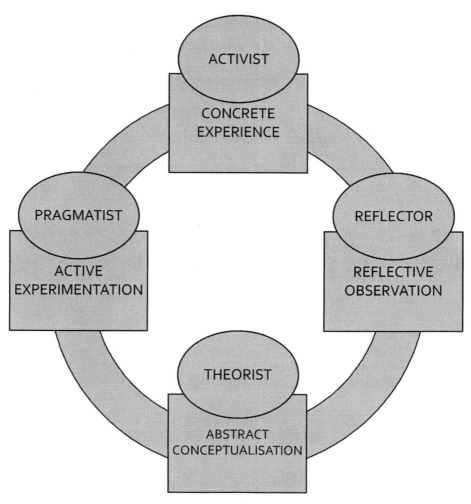

Figure 10.2: Honey and Mumford learner types[3]

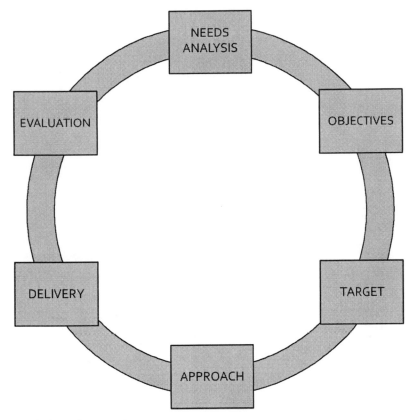

Figure 10.3: Learning event process

Learning event planning

Understanding how to design a learning event is crucial if we are to successfully educate participants. Learning events may vary in size from an individual to a lecture theatre full of participants. No matter the size or setting of the learning event the basic framework for the event remains the same. The framework of a learning event may be considered as a process comprising of a number of key stages (*see* Figure 10.3).

These stages are as follows.

➤ Needs assessment.
➤ Objectives.
➤ Target audience.
➤ Approach.
➤ Delivery.
➤ Evaluation.

Needs assessment

The initial stage provides the information necessary to design our learning event. Analysis of the organisation, requirements, knowledge, skills and abilities form the basis of the stage.

Organisational analysis

Organisational analysis is concerned with examination of organisational goals, resources, climate for training, and internal and external constraints present in the environment.[4] This is an important part of our first stage and it is essential to develop a supportive relationship with top-level divisional management in order to gain time, effort and financial support for such an event.

Learning organisations

Senge[5] described the learning organisation as:

> *... organisations where people continually expand their capacity to create the results they truly desire, where new and expansive patterns of thinking are nurtured, where collective aspiration is set free, and where people are continually learning to see the whole together.*

Senge identifies five learning disciplines to building a learning organisation. These are as follows.

➤ **Personal mastery** – This is the discipline of continual personal development through commitment to learning.
➤ **Mental models** – These are deeply ingrained assumptions, generalisations, or even pictures and images that influence how we understand the world and how we take action.
➤ **Building shared vision** – A shared vision of future direction that is inspirational to an organisation is instrumental to motivate its achievement.
➤ **Team learning** – It is suggested that better results and more rapid growth occur when teams learn together as opposed to individuals.
➤ **Systems thinking** – This is the fifth discipline that integrates the previous four and describes their interaction with one another.

Requirements analysis

What do we need for the learning event?

This analysis explores the necessary facilities and resources required for the learning event to take place.

Knowledge, skill and ability (KSA) analysis

What knowledge, skills and abilities are we trying to teach during this event? Prien defined knowledge, skills and abilities as follows.[4]

➤ **Knowledge** – refers to an organised body of knowledge, usually of a factual or procedural nature, which, if applied, makes adequate job performance possible. It should be noted that possession of knowledge does not ensure that it will be used. Therefore it is important that appropriate application of knowledge is also taught.
➤ **Skill** – refers to the capability to perform job operations with ease and precision. The specification of a skill implies a performance standard that is usually required for effective job operations.

➤ **Ability** – refers to cognitive capabilities necessary to perform a job function. Most often abilities require the application of some knowledge base.

Person analysis
The final step in determining training needs focuses on the individual employees or participants. It identifies where and what training is required.

Objectives

Learning objectives or outcomes define the attitudinal, behavioural or performance outcomes that are to be achieved. Final behavioural objectives are the outcomes the learner should have achieved once the learning event is complete. Interim behavioural objectives are outcomes achieved at each key stage of the learning process.[6] Learning objectives should be carefully defined to be appropriate, realistic, achievable and measurable.

Target audience

Who are we teaching?

The target audience of learning event needs to be well defined. This should be based largely on the basis of the analyses undertaken in the previous stage. When we have defined the target audience, it allows the event to be tailored more closely to their needs. The target audience also defines our target market to promote the event to.

Approach

How will the learning be presented?

The way the event is presented again relies on the analyses stage. The approaches are highly dependent on the task, knowledge, skill or ability that is being taught during the event. In some circumstances, a lecture-based approach may be more appropriate in comparison with a small group setting. In medicine, case-based discussions and problem-based learning techniques may be useful. Advances in technology have also enhanced online learning approaches.

Lectures
Lectures are a highly efficient method of delivering information to a large group of students. This method of delivery is not, however, the most effective.[7] The lecture setting often promotes more passive learning and student often feel it is an opportunity to learn by osmosis. This can be improved by providing more interaction with the audience, which can be in the form of asking questions or being asked questions. The presentation should be well illustrated with examples or media to keep the audience engaged. Provision of handouts will also allow students to listen and reflect on what they are being taught rather than frantically making notes.

Small group
Small group teaching allows closer contact between the teacher and students. In this setting students should feel more comfortable expressing their ideas and thoughts. It also provides an opportunity to work in a team and develop communication

skills. In medical education, there has been a move more towards this form of teaching method. Specific forms of small group teaching include case or problem based learning sessions.

Case and problem-based learning

Problem-based learning (PBL) is an approach that uses cases or scenarios to allow student orientated learning in a small group setting.[8] This method of learning encourages students to take responsibility for their learning, direct the process and collaborate with each other. The teacher facilitates the group by providing guidance, encouraging participation by all students, time keeping, assessing and ensuring objectives are met. The group appoints a chairperson who leads the group in its discussions. Additionally, a scribe may be allocated to keep records of the discussions. The University of Maastricht described the 'seven jump step' model for the PBL process, which is outlined below (*see* Figure 10.4).[9]

➤ **Clarification** – The chair presents the case or scenario to the group. Clarification of any unfamiliar terms used in the case are discussed and noted.
➤ **Problem identification** – The group agrees the issues or problems arising from the scenario and the scribe records these.
➤ **Brainstorm** – The group discusses these problems and draws from their prior knowledge in providing explanations. Areas of knowledge deficit are identified and recorded.
➤ **Review** – The scribe and chair review the problem identification and brainstorm steps.
➤ **Learning objectives** – The group formulates and agrees the learning objectives. The teacher ensures the objectives are appropriate and achievable.
➤ **Private study** – The students collect information and knowledge relating to the learning objectives.
➤ **Group discussion** – The group reconvenes to discuss the learning objectives and their newfound knowledge. The teacher ensures the objectives are met and may take an opportunity to assess the students.

Case-based learning is similar to PBL but the former provides a more guided and more structured method of teaching.[10]

Simulation

The role of simulation-based training is becoming more prevalent in medicine. Simulation-based training models can vary greatly in complexity from basic cannula models to live animal models. A significant amount of research has been undertaken investigating the effectiveness of simulation-based learning. Most of the evidence suggests that this is a valid and good method of teaching specific skills in a number of specialties and scenarios.

E-learning

The internet provides a wealth of information which is readily accessible. Technology has also allowed enhanced interactivity between users over the internet. Consequently, the internet has become a further method of learning which has

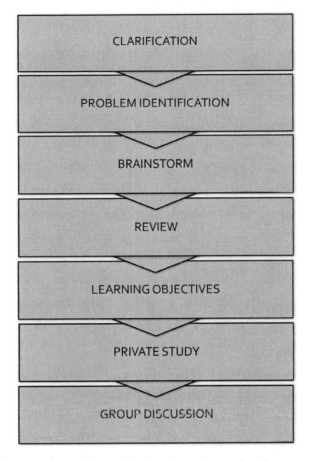

Figure 10.4: The seven-jump step model for problem-based learning

been adopted by many established learning institutions. The amount of reliance on web-based learning platforms varies depending on the course and institution. Some courses are completely distance learning based with no face-to-face contact whilst others use e-learning as an adjunct to conventional methods. The content of e-learning courses can vary greatly from additional reading materials to full virtual learning environments (VLE). VLE provide students with a interactive site that typically contain reading materials, videos, lectures, administrative information, assessment tools, discussion forums and student interaction platforms such as chat rooms.[11]

Delivery

This is the actual delivery of the event. What will be the structure of the day and timetable?

The logistics for the training event need to be considered. Part of the delivery plan should include time required to set up special equipment and ensuring all presentations are functioning properly.

Evaluation

Evaluation of the learning event is an important stage of the overall process. This stage determines the success of the event in delivering its objectives and meeting the needs of the participants. The evaluation process provides feedback to both participants and trainers on their performance during the event. This stage also identifies strengths and weaknesses of the event and provides information for further developing the event. To help identify factors for evaluation Warr[12] devised the CIRO framework. This framework describes four dimensions: context in which the learning event has taken place; inputs; reactions; and outcomes.

Context

This involves establishing how accurately we diagnosed the needs, why the course was introduced, the rationale for purpose and objectives, and organisational support given by managers and the workplace. This analysis helps identify strengths and weaknesses of the course.[6]

Inputs

This dimension investigates the cost associated with the course. Opportunity costs, in terms of off-the-job time, by trainers and trainees must also be considered. The profitability of the course and allocation of resources must be considered during this stage.

Reactions to the learning event

This involves discovering the trainees' perceptions of the course, and explores the delivery and content of the event. We know that these perceptions are important in determining the expectations and performance of future participants.

Outcomes of the learning event

The outcomes of course may be analysed on a number of levels including the learner, workplace, unit and organisational levels. Validation at a learner level may be achieved by trainee assessment. Workplace level outcome measures may be assessed using appraisals or observations. We can also assess changes at a unit level to see if performance has improved following a learning event.

Summary

Learning and teaching are an important component of medicine. A basic understanding of learning theory is useful for any teacher. When planning a learning event one must consider many different aspects to ensure an effective and efficient event that meets the needs of its participants. The framework described here should form a useful foundation to build a learning event upon.

Exercises

1 Consider a task that you would like to teach someone. Can you define the knowledge, skills and abilities you are trying to teach?
2 Think of the different types of learning scenarios you have been involved in, such as lectures, small groups, simulations or PBLs. Which did you find most effective and why?
3 Design a training event using the structured framework covered in this module.

Sample answer for training event

Microsurgical techniques are becoming increasingly popular in plastic surgical practice. The purpose of this event is to develop a two-day introductory microsurgery course.

Needs assessment

Organisational analysis

This course provides ensure junior staff with the necessary knowledge and skills to develop microsurgical skills. The department and consultants who will assist in the running of the course support this. Funding is provided by donations to the departmental research fundRequirements analysis

The course will be undertaken in our department using training microscopes on loan from the company that manufactures them.

KSA analysis

The table below summarises some of the knowledge, skills and abilities to be developed during this course.

KSAs
Knowledge of microsurgical instruments
Knowledge of the microscope and its settings
Knowledge of steps used in nerve and vessel repair
Ability to organise instruments in preparation for a procedure
Ability to recognise differences and similarities between normal suturing and microsurgical suturing
Ability to recognise the steps in microsurgical repair and assist accordingly
Skills in the use of the microscope
Skills in the handling of microsurgical instruments
Skills in performing suturing using a microscope and micro-instruments
Skills in performing a nerve repair using microsurgical techniques
Skills in performing a vessel anastomosis using microsurgical techniques

Objectives

The primary learning outcomes of this course are to provide intellectual skills for the use of the microscope and instruments and also, to teach motor skills in microsurgical techniques.

Target audience

These trainees will consist mainly of junior members of the team with little or no microsurgical experience. This microsurgical course will have a faculty of four tutors and this should allow eight trainees to participate on the course.

Approach

The first day of the event commences with the introduction of the faculty. During the introductions, the new trainees are expected to provide details about their level of training and experience. Trainees are also asked why they are attending and what they expect from the course. The faculty demonstrates the microscope and how it is used. The trainees are then asked to perform a simple zooming and focusing task. The faculty proceeds to the introduction of the microsurgical instruments. The trainees are then given an opportunity to use these instruments. They are then given an opportunity to place sutures in a simulated scar in a latex glove using the microscope. The tutors observe the trainees and provide feedback on their performance.

A demonstration of a nerve repair is then shown to the trainees. The tutor points out the key steps in performing the procedure. Trainees are then allowed to perform this task using a chicken leg. Tutors again review performance and provide feedback.

Day 2 consists of a live demonstration and practice of vessel anastomosis using a chicken leg model. The day closes with trainee evaluation of the course and feedback from the tutors regarding changes in assessment scores during the course.

Evaluation

Feedback from the course participants is collected to allow for course improvement and development. The participants are given feedback on performance using validated assessment tools used in microsurgery. We can also assess if the learning objectives outlined have been achieved.

References

1 Kolb D. *Experiential Learning: Experience as the Source of Learning and Development.* Englewood Cliffs, NJ: Prentice Hall; 1984.
2 Kolb DA. Management and the learning process. *California Management Review.* 1976; **18**: 21–31.
3 Honey P, Mumford A. *The Manual of Learning Styles.* Maidenhead: Honey, Ardingly House; 1992.
4 Goldstein IL, Ford JK. *Training in Organizations.* 4th ed. Belmont, CA: Wadsworth; 2002.
5 Senge PM. *The Fifth Discipline: The Art and Practice of the Learning Organization.* New York: Doubleday; 2006.
6 Harrison R. *Learning and Development.* 4th ed. London: CIPD; 2006.
7 Cantillon P. ABC of learning and teaching: Teaching large groups. *British Medical Journal.* 2003; **326**: 437.
8 Wood DF. ABC of learning and teaching: Problem based learning. *British Medical Journal.* 2003; **326**: 328–30.
9 Wilkerson L, Gijselaers WH. *Bringing Problem-Based Learning to Higher Education: Theory and Practice. New Directions for Teaching and Learning.* San Francisco, CA: Jossey-Bass Publishers; 1996.
10 Srinivasan M, Wilkes M, Stevenson F, *et al.* Comparing problem-based learning with case-based learning: effects of a major curricular shift at two institutions. *Academic Medicine.* 2007; **82**: 74–82.
11 McKimm J, Jollie C, Cantillon P. ABC of learning and teaching: web based learning. *British Medical Journal.* 2003; **326**: 870–3.
12 Warr P, Bird MW, Rackham N. *Evaluation of Management Training.* Aldershot: Gower; 1970.

Further reading

➤ Harrison R. *Learning and Development.* 4th ed. London: CIPD; 2006.

Useful websites

Chartered Institute of Personnel and Development: www.cipd.co.uk/subjects/lrnand dev/
NHS Connecting for Health – e-learning: www.connectingforhealth.nhs.uk/systemsand services/etd/elearning

Coping with change in the clinical environment

Change management

Change may be considered as a transition from a current state to a future desired state.

There are varying drivers or sources of change, which include the following.

➤ **Change for service improvement** – Changes to how a service is delivered.
➤ **Organisational change** – Restructuring, reorganisation.
➤ **Change for development** – Promotions.

Within the healthcare setting, we are seeing many changes in terms of technology, organisation, management, politics and economics. It is therefore important that we have a good grasp of effective change management to facilitate these changes.

Change management involves exploration of three main aspects (*see* Figure 11.1):

➤ People.
➤ Organisational culture.
➤ Processes.

We shall explore these in turn and then investigate why some change initiatives fail before discussing methods for successful change.

People

People are crucial in any change management initiative. We must understand the feelings experienced when faced with change and learn methods to assist people to accept change.

Stages of change

Being clinicians, we should be familiar with the Kubler-Ross model for the stages of grief. This model provides the basis for the stages of transition seen in change. In 1969, Kubler-Ross described the process, consisting of five stages, by which people deal with tragedy or grief (*see* Figure 11.2).[1] Although these stages were originally

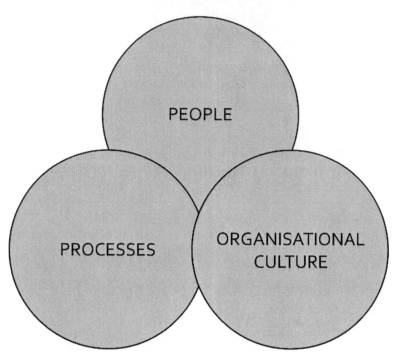

Figure 11.1: Change management

described for terminal illness it can be seen they can be applied to other situations. These situations can include the diagnosis of illness, significant life event or loss. The stages of the process include the following.

➤ **Denial** – The patient refuses believe or accept the fact initially. This is usually only a temporary defence mechanism. Following the initial denial, there may be anxiety and concern about coping.

➤ **Anger** – The patient begins to realise that denial can no longer continue. An expression of anger ensues and this can make the person difficult to care for.

➤ **Bargaining** – This stage involves bargaining and hope to delay the end result. Negotiation for this delay is often made with positions of power that can impact the quality of their life or higher powers. Bargaining often involves offering certain changes in lifestyle to delay their death.

➤ **Depression** – The patient realises the inevitable certainty of their death. During this stage, the patient becomes withdrawn and distant sinking into depression.

➤ **Acceptance** – The patient becomes resigned to their fate and will slowly climb out of 'the valley of despair'. They accept the inevitable and try their utmost to move on with their lives.

This model provides a good basis for understanding how people deal with change. On an individual basis there are a number of factors influencing any resistance to change, including the following.

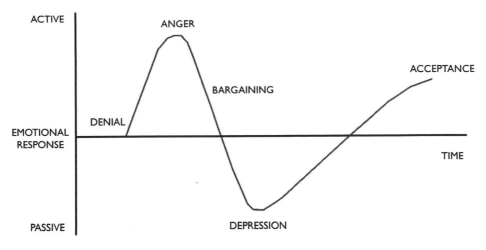

Figure 11.2: Kubler-Ross stages of grief[1]

> **They haven't participated in the change** – When management pushes initiatives through without inviting feedback from those affected, there is no sense of 'owning the change'.
> **They don't believe the change is possible** – People become cynical and disillusioned when they recall past changes that were not supported.
> **They don't see the change as being in their best interest** – When people can't see how the change will benefit them, they won't back the process.
> **They maintain allegiance to the status quo or habit** – People like change but hate to be changed. Doing a job the same way every day is easy; learning a new set of steps isn't. For the same pay, most people prefer not to have to deal with anything new.
> **They fear the unknown** – Employees become used to their boss, their job, and relationships with others within the organisation. A disruption in these familiar patterns may create anxiety because it can cause delays and give rise to the belief that nothing is getting accomplished.

Changes can also create a situation described as *'quicksand'* – people become so overwhelmed by various change programmes happening within the same organisation all at the same time.

Organisational culture

Organisational culture is a system of shared meaning held by members that distinguishes the organisation from other organisations.[2] The culture of an organisation may be appraised by seven characteristics (*see* Figure 11.3). Large organisations have a dominant culture that expresses the core values that are shared by a majority of the organisation's members. Subcultures may, however, develop that include the core values with additional values unique to them. In a strong culture, the organisation's core values are intensely held and widely accepted.[2] Organisational culture determines the codes of conduct within an organisation whilst making employees feel like they belong to the company.

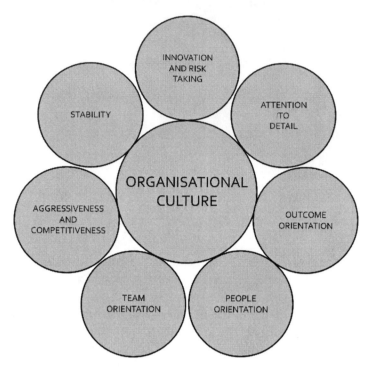

Figure 11.3: Characteristics of organisational culture

We have already seen reasons for resistance to change on an individual level. Resistance can also occur at an organisational level and the underlying reasons include the following.

> **Structural inertia** – Organisational culture determines persons selected to 'fit' into the organisation. Change results in disruption of this stability.
> **Limited focus of change** – Changes need to be implemented across the organisation's departments, which are related. Changing one will have an impact on other departments and this must be considered.
> **Group inertia** – Group norms can act as a constraint even if some individuals are willing to change. If the group as a whole is resistant it is unlikely an individual will go against them.
> **Threat to expertise** – Changes may threaten specialist experts by depowering them.
> **Threat to established power relationships** – Changes in the decision-making authority can threaten power relationship that has been developed into the organisational culture.
> **Threat to established resource allocations** – Change can threaten staffing and resource allocations. In view of this there can be strong resistance against change.

Processes

Understanding processes and their improvement is an integral part of change management. During the operations management module, we reviewed a number of process improvement techniques such as Six Sigma, Lean and process re-engineering. Refer to this module for further details regarding process improvement and implementation.

Why does change fail?

Every company, big or small, would like to change for the better. But is positive change really attainable? Moreover, can it be made relatively painless?
Before you answer, consider the following four demoralising facts:

➤ Eighty-five percent of Fortune 1000 companies have downsized workforces in the past five years, but their overhead rates remain significantly above the best global competitors.
➤ Hundreds of organisations in the United States have undertaken major restructurings, but 52% of executives surveyed say these efforts have not met original targets.
➤ Billions have been spent to automate inefficient business processes, but information systems have proven to be among the least effective at improving productivity because most of the time organisations simply go out and buy equipment to install without taking into consideration other pertinent factors affecting productivity. The bigger the problem, the bigger the sum of money spent on buying hardware. But money spent will be wasted if organisations think that buying the newest and the fastest equipment is the solution to their problems. Organisations should also consider if their people are ready for radical change, if new equipment is the answer and if there is sufficient change management initiatives to cushion the impact of change.
➤ Hundreds of major corporations have made acquisitions to build synergies by purchasing equipment which they think will integrate various departments of the corporations together, but only one in three investments has generated a return greater than the buyer's cost of capital.

Seven out of 10 management initiatives fail – not because they're bad ideas, but because they aren't properly implemented and sustained. The downsizers mentioned above failed because their focus was on getting rid of people, not on changing the remaining staff's behaviour and business processes. The reformers failed because they concentrated on the organisation's structure, not on people and what they do. The big spenders intent on improving efficiency failed because they focused on technology, not on the people applying it. And the would-be synergisers failed because they concentrated on integrating plants rather than people.[3]

Leading a successful change initiative

So what does it take to lead and manage a successful change initiative? How can all the individuals, groups, organisations and business processes involved become properly aligned? Here are some possible solutions.

➤ **Education and communication** – If employee resistance is based on inaccurate or inadequate information, set up a programme to communicate the details of the change.

➤ **Participation and involvement** – You can reduce resistance to change by involving those who will be affected in shaping it – this should include patients. How are the changes you are implementing going to affect them?

➤ **Facilitation and support** – When employees are having difficulty in adjusting to new arrangements and ways of doing things, you may need to provide additional training or extra emotional support until everyone is accustomed to the system.

➤ **Negotiation and agreement** – If certain people or groups are losing something significant because of the change and have enough power to resist it strongly (as a union in a hospital might), senior management may want to negotiate. Negotiation before implementation can make the change go much more smoothly.

➤ **Manipulation and cooptation** – In situations where other methods do not work or cannot be used, senior management may resort to manipulating information, resources and favours to overcome resistance. Electing representatives of groups likely to offer resistance to a group or committee – in other words, cooptation – may be a way of defusing the situation by including them in the design and implementation of change. Make your enemies your friends.

➤ **Coercion** – Senior management may resort to coercion – threats of pay reduction, demotion, transfer or dismissal – to overcome resistance if all other methods fail. While this may be a quick method of overcoming opposition, it can seriously affect employee attitudes and have adverse consequences in the long run.

Kotter,[4] in his book *Leading Change*, described an eight-stage process for successful change implementation (*see* Figure 11.4).

➤ **Establish a sense of urgency** – Motivate and inspire to get the process off the ground. Highlight the reasons for change and why these are required promptly, such as competitors producing new product.

➤ **Creating the guiding coalition** – Create a driving team for change. Develop a team of individuals with their own strengths who share the desire for change. The team must express the need for change and inspire motivation for this change.

➤ **Developing a vision and strategy** – What is the vision for the change process? How are we going to achieve this?

➤ **Communicating the change vision** – The vision must be regularly communicated across the organisation. Keep the message simple and involve as many people as possible. Understand the concerns and needs of people respond to them.

➤ **Empowering employees and removing obstacles** – Allow people to express themselves and become involved in the process. Remove obstacles to change. Identify people resisting change and help them appreciate the need for change. Recognise and reward those who have helped implement change.

➤ **Generating short-term wins** – Create intermediate goals that are readily achievable. Completion of each goal is recognised and rewarded.

➤ **Consolidating gains and producing more change** – Explore success and the reasons for it. Investigate how things could be improved further. Set more goals based on the momentum that has been built up already.

➤ **Anchoring new approaches in the corporate culture** – The change must become part of the organisational culture. Employ people who 'fit' the successful change process. Promote successful change agents.

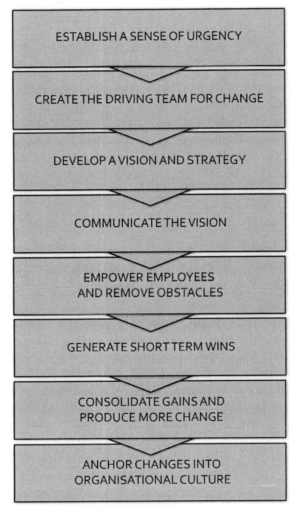

Figure 11.4: Kotter's eight-stage process for change implementation[4]

Summary

Change is important for any organisation. We have seen that when considering change we must look at the people, culture and processes of an organisation. We have identified some reasons for resistance to change at the individual and organisational level. We have also reviewed useful methods for successfully implementing change into an organisation.

Exercises

1   In your environment, what do you see are the major drivers of change? Which one has the greatest impact on the patient experience?
2   What if change is inevitable but yet you fear that some pockets of the people impacted may not be ready for change. What would you do?
3   Identify some reasons why people and organisations resist change and suggest ways to overcome their resistance.
4   As a clinician, how can you demonstrate your willingness to embrace and champion change?

References

1   Kubler-Ross E. *On Death and Dying*. Abingdon: Routledge; 1973.
2   Robbins SP. *Organisational Behaviour*. 10th ed. Saddle River, NJ: Prentice Hall; 2003.
3   Loh M. *Re-engineering at Work*. Aldershot: Gower; 1997.
4   Kotter JP. *Leading Change*. Boston, MA: Harvard Business School Press; 1996.

Further reading

➤   Kotter JP. *Leading Change*. Boston, MA: Harvard Business School Press; 1996.

Useful websites

NHS Connecting for Health – Change Management: www.connectingforhealth.nhs.uk/ systemsandservices/capability/phi/personal/learningweb/leadership/change

Innovation in medicine

Innovation is defined as the introduction of new ideas and processes. In medicine, it is about thinking and applying knowledge to the practice of medicine. It is about thinking outside the box, to create new ideas, invent new materials, instruments and processes for the ultimate benefit of the patient.

What today's undergraduate curriculum, postgraduate training and the risk-averse clinical environment have done is produce practicing clinicians who have great resistance to being innovative. The obsession with performance delivery by healthcare agencies and control and punitive actions by regulators has also compounded the issue.

In 2003, Zlotnik-Shaul and McKneall[1] stated that:

> ... the ethical imperative to improve practice through innovation and research finds justification in the requirements of the doctors to help patients, minimise harm and disease, and to bring the benefits of scientific medicine to patients.

The very foundation of medical practice is to innovate. Even the regulatory body in the United Kingdom, in its requirements of good medical practice states that doctors must work with colleagues to monitor, maintain and improve the quality of care provided. Innovation is the thus part and parcel of good medical practice.

All healthcare organisations must provide an environment that is conducive to innovation. The areas in healthcare are where innovation is possible include organisational, technological, product and service sectors. The degree of novelty those innovations display can vary from radical innovations to more minor or incremental innovations possibly resulting from a simple adaptation or change. Thus innovation must be considered subjectively, and in relative rather than in absolute terms.[2]

The delivery of healthcare is a team effort, and it is therefore obvious that areas for innovation require a team approach. Rosenberg showed that interdisciplinary research would benefit healthcare agencies.[3] The Anglo-American experience suggests the great value of locating medical research and medical education inside an academic community. A great strength of the US academic medical centres is that they have vastly facilitated interdisciplinary research, along two dimensions: (1) much greater opportunities for joint research, such as between medical schools, on the one hand, and physics and electrical engineering, on the other; and (2) they brought together, under the same roof, clinicians and scientific disciplines that were becoming more directly relevant to the medical world. So the evidence and expectation of regulators is that innovation is possible and an imperative part of medical practice. This is a paradigm shift for doctors who are expected not to be inventive or innovative and stick to old ways.

The innovative healthcare organisation

Innovation must start from the top and diffuse down throughout the organisation. From the top this corporate culture must trickle down to the middle managers, the frontline supervisors and finally the frontline staff to be innovative. The chief executive must be innovative and this must be known amongst the rest of the organisation. If the chief executive wants the frontline staff to deliver innovative care and service, then they need the help and passion of their top-level management. The management should provide all that is necessary for the frontline staff to do just that. This must be made known to the front line. The author recollects a discussion with the deputy chief executive of his NHS organisation who told me that if I needed an item to improve my delivery of service just let him know, for if I was successful as a doctor he will take credit for making the environment conducive for me to succeed. This is a typical win-win scenario.

In healthcare it is the frontline staff who deliver the service and care and they are owners of the service processes. So who better than the front-liners to innovate healthcare? Innovation has to be become part of their job descriptions. In the United Kingdom, the incentive schemes for doctors, such as Clinical Excellence Awards, include the innovative delivery of services as part of the evaluation criteria in awarding points, which translates to monetary rewards.

Frontline staff must be clear what the corporate mission is for their healthcare organisation. It has to become the daily mantra so that they are constantly reminded of it. Once they can see this they will be able to explore how innovation can be applied and be aligned to the corporate objectives of the organisation.

How does management need to work to ensure these innovations happen from the frontline staff?

The management needs to understand that their very existence is to ensure frontline staff can work effectively – the front-liners are their employees. Below are some useful tips for managers.

1 Be accessible to the front-liners.
2 Listen to them and engage their views, however ridiculous.
3 Give them what they want to deliver the service.
4 Enable them with the infrastructure and services, to deliver their service.
5 Don't punish mistakes – support them and let the front-liners know this! Celebrate failure!

Peters and Waterman[4] observe in their book:

> ... the perfect failure concept arises from [the] simple recognition that all research and development is inherently risky, that the only way to succeed at

all is through lots of tries, that management's primary objective should be to induce lots of tries, and that a good try that results in some learning is to be celebrated even when it fails.

The frontline staff must be reassured that if they make honest mistakes, they will not be merely tolerated but will be vigorously defended and that those in the organisation who are willing to experiment with innovative ways to improve performance will be protected, even at personal cost to the management.[5]

The innovative management

How can management encourage innovation?

➤ Create job descriptions that include the need to be innovative and **include innovation in the key performance indicators** of doctors. Individual innovations must contribute to achieving the organisation's purposes. They must be achieving quality and improvement in care delivered to patients directly or indirectly. In the job plan include multiple roles and multi-tasking so that doctors can see the whole picture of their complex organisation and create opportunities to innovate. A nurse can observe and look at an innovative way of doing a particular process that a doctor performs or vice versa.

➤ The organisations producing more innovation have more complex structures that link people in multiple ways and encourage them to 'do what needs to be done' within strategically guided limits (mission and goals), rather than confining themselves to the letter of their job.[6]

➤ **Don't reward individuals but teams** and move towards team appraisal. Rewards need not be monetary and managers need to be innovative on how to reward teams.

➤ **Change the organisation structure** to a flat one with the ownership and empowerment to the strategic clinical unit (SCU). The SCU is discussed in further detail in the clinical team module. Give the SCU what it needs and ensure some finance and procurement members of management answer to the team! Management must provide all the necessary resources especially information for this SCU to function and deliver on innovation.

The innovative doctor

On an individual level, to be innovative doctors need to do the following.

➤ **Know your patients well, the way they the use the service and what their fears and concerns are** – Your practice exists for them and them alone. Understanding your patient is crucial if you want to make an impact on your patient with your innovation. I remember more than 20 years ago when we introduced day surgery practice in Malaysia, we found that patients were fearful of going home after surgery on the same day. So we introduced a service of calling all patients who had day surgery in the evening to check on them and this greatly improved the patient experience.

➤ **Think outside the box** – Look at other industries and processes and think how you can apply them to your practice. Visit other services, read journals and magazines not related to healthcare. It is amazing how easily you can transfer ideas from one service to another. Hopefully, this is becoming more apparent as you progress through this book.

➤ **Celebrate and embrace problems** – They are opportunity for innovations. Identify problems comprehensively and the solutions will be in the problem.

➤ **Make innovation an important part of your practice** – It has to be part of your good medical practice. Know your clinical processes well. Methods of process improvement can be used and these are discussed further in the operations module.

➤ **Network with others** who may help you look at your challenges then provide solutions. Look at other professionals who can provide expertise. Collaborate with others. Innovate collaboration – have a tea party for potential collaborators and present your clinical challenges – you will be surprised at what they may have to offer. Masters students in university are always looking for practical and real-life solutions where they can apply their academia. Register for free at www.researchgate.net/ – where you will have more than 200,000 scientists at your disposal. ResearchGate is a free, web-based portal which seeks to improve scientific collaboration and the exchange of ideas across the world. The solution gives scientists the power to interact and collaborate with researchers from a variety of different fields.

➤ **Take risks** – Yes, take risks and celebrate your failures. Nothing worthwhile came out of being risk averse and towing the line. It is difficult when you have been trained not to be innovative. But what if you shift your paradigm and look at good medical practice afresh – it has to be what is best for the patient. You need to try new things so that you can do what is best for your patient. Jaideep Prabhu, of the Judge Business School, Cambridge, says that the rule in pharmaceuticals – one in five molecules make it to market –also applies to other sectors. 'Even then, one in three products is likely to fail after launch.'

➤ **Look to the future** – See what is happening. I now regularly subscribe to technology journals as I am always looking for new technology and processes to see how they can be applied to the healthcare sector.

➤ **Keep improving always** – See how you can always improve – ask others how something could be done better, what new technology can be applied for better use of resources.

➤ **Dream the impossible** – Forget what cannot be done but think of what is possible. It all starts with a dream, so dream your innovation and get others to dream also. Try and reinvent medicine as you see it.

Innovation can be and is fun.

Exercises

1 Identify a product, person or process in your practice that you have considered to be innovative. Why did you think it was innovative? Did it improve effectiveness or efficiency? Did others feel the same?
2 Think of an innovative process or product. Did you embrace or resist its use? Why did you embrace or resist it?
3 What measures can you take to encourage people to more readily embrace innovation?

References

1 Zlotnik-Shaul R, McKneally MF. Ethical considerations for innovations and clinical trials. *Seminars in Thoracic and Cardiovascular Surgery.* 2003; **15**(4): 380–5.
2 Djellal F, Gallouj F. Mapping innovation dynamics in hospitals. *Research Policy.* 2005; **34**(6): 817–35.
3 Rosenberg N. Some critical episodes in the progress of medical innovation: an Anglo-American perspective. *Research Policy.* 2009; **38**(2): 234–42.
4 Peters TJ, Waterman RH. *In Search of Excellence: Lessons from America's Best-run Companies.* New York: Harper & Row; 1982.
5 Behn R. Creating an innovative organisation: ten hints for involving frontline workers. *State and Local Government Review.* 1995; **27**(3): 221–34.
6 Kanter RM. When a thousand flowers bloom: structural, collective, and social conditions for innovation in organisations. *Organisational Behavior.* 1988; **10**: 169–211.

Further reading

➤ Drucker PF. *Innovation and Entrepreneurship.* Oxford: Butterworth-Heinemann; 2007.

Useful websites

NHS Institute for Innovation and Improvement: www.institute.nhs.uk/innovation/innovation/introduction.html
ResearchGate: www.researchgate.net/

Glossary

Accounting – the system of making records, verifications and reporting of the value of assets, liabilities, expenses and income in the account books.

Ansoff product-growth matrix – a useful tool for devising growth strategies for an organisation based on its products or services, and new or existing markets.

Assets – are the rights and things that a company owns. They can be either current or fixed assets. Current assets include stock, cash, and trade debtors (money owed to you). Fixed assets may be classified into tangible and intangible. Tangible fixed assets include land, property, machinery and vehicles. Intangible fixed assets are things such as goodwill, patents, copyrights and brands an organisation may possess.

Balance sheet – statement of assets and liabilities at the end of the accounting period (a 'snapshot') of the business.

Cash flow statement – the cash inflows and outflows during the accounting period.

Change – a transition from a current state to a future desired state.

Clinical team – a group of clinicians working collectively for the common goal of improving the patient outcome from a clinical episode.

Coaching – a process whereby an individual, through direct discussion and guided activity, helps a colleague to learn to solve a problem, or to do a task, better than would otherwise be the case over a short term.

Conflict – any process caused by someone that may be perceived by someone else as negatively affecting something they care about.

Cost leadership – ensuring a firm delivers a product or service at the lowest possible cost to them.

Culture – is a system of shared meaning and beliefs held by members that distinguishes the organisation from other organisations.

Delegation – distributing responsibility for tasks to other members of an organisation or team.

Dependability – provision or delivery of services or products to the customer exactly when they were promised them.

Effectiveness – the extent to which a goal is met.

Efficiency – the achievement of a goal in an economical and timely manner.

Equity – the cash invested into the company by its owners or shareholders.

Fixed costs – costs incurred over a period irrespective of the level of output or resources used.

Flexibility – the ability of the operation to be changed.

Innovation – the introduction of new ideas and processes.

Job enlargement – expanding the number of different tasks performed by broadening the scope of the job.

Job enrichment – giving employees responsibility for the planning, organisation, control and evaluation of the job.

Key performance indicators – quantifiable measurements, agreed beforehand by the doctor and the management, that reflect the critical success factors of the healthcare organisation.

Lean – a method of process improvement by eliminating waste.

Lean Six Sigma – process improvement using a combination of Lean and Six Sigma.

Liabilities – borrowings the company owes.

Management – the organisational process that involves managing resources, inclusive of human and financial assets, needed to achieve the objectives of the organisation, and monitoring the outcomes.

Market segmentation – identification and division of the target market into distinct groups or segments.

Marketing – the activity, set of institutions and processes for creating, communicating, delivering and exchanging offerings that have value for customers, clients, partners and society at large.

Marketing mix – a set of controllable, tactical marketing tools that work together to achieve a company's objectives.

Maslow's hierarchy of needs – five needs exist: physiological, safety, social, esteem and self-actualisation

Mentoring – a process whereby senior employees provide guidance and direction to less experienced members of the team over a more long-term period.

Operations management – managing all the activities required to create and deliver your goods or services, measurement and analysis of processes, and methods of improving the performance.

Opportunity costs – opportunities that were not pursued in favour of the chosen product or service.

Organisational culture – a system of shared meaning held by members that distinguishes the organisation from other organisations.

Performance – how well the patient pathway is managed and the value delivered to the patient, the clinical team and the community in utilising resources efficiently and effectively.

PESTEL – a method of analysing the macro-environment around an organisation. Components are: Political, Economic, Social, Technological, Environmental and Legal.

Porter's five forces – five major forces that determine the state of competition in a particular industry or sector: threat of entry, threat of substitutes, power of suppliers, power of buyers and competitive rivalry.

Porter's strategies – three main generic strategies an organisation may develop: cost leadership, differentiation and focus.

Profit and loss account – the trading performance of the business over the accounting period.

Process re-engineering – fundamentally rethinking and redesigning processes to obtain dramatic and sustaining improvements in quality, cost, service, lead-times, outcomes, flexibility and innovation.

Product life cycle – defines the stages of a product's life, which include: development, introduction, growth, maturity and decline.

Quality – ensuring things are done correctly. Characterised by functionality, appearance, reliability, durability and contact.

Six Sigma – a method of process improvement by reducing variation in a process by using the stages: Define, Measure, Analyse, Improve and Control (DMAIC).

SMART objectives – Specific, Measurable, Agreed, Realistic, Time-based.

Speed – the period of time from customer request to delivery of product and service.

Strategic clinical unit – the core team involved in the provision and delivery of care to that patient.

Strategic human resource management – numerous activities related to the management of these employees, which include: workforce planning, recruitment, rewards, retention, teamwork, training and appraisal.

Strategy – process of pursuing a vision and planning how to achieve it.

Sunk costs – costs that have been incurred that cannot be recovered.

SWOT – a method of analysis employed in strategic planning: Strengths, Weaknesses, Opportunities and Threats.

Turnover – when employees leave a job and need to be replaced.

Variable costs – costs that vary depending on the level of activity.

Workforce planning – the designing, development and delivery of the workforce.

Index

ability 107
absenteeism 64
abstract conceptualisation 102, 103
academic literature 56, 57
academic sector 29
acceptance of change 116
accountability 78, 91
accounting and finance 5–12
  accounting formula 6–8
  anatomy of management 2
  balance sheet 8–9
  case study 8
  cash flow statement 10–11
  company law requirements 6
  definition of accounting 5, 128
  definition of finance 5–6
  profit and loss account 9–10
  ratio analysis 11–12
Accounting Standards 6
accreditation 94
acid-ratio 11
active experimentation 102, 103
activist learning style 104
adjourning stage of team development 72
adult learning theory 104
Advanced Life Support 72
advertising 3, 32, 35, 36, 64
advocates 35, 36
affluents 35, 36
age discrimination 47
Alred, G 87
American Marketing Association 28, 41
American Medical Association (AMA) 92, 93, 101
American Society for Quality 27
analysis for strategic management 43
anger 116
annual accounts 6
ANSI X12 (EDI) 55
Ansoff product-growth matrix 36, 49–50, 128

appraisal 93, 97, 125
The Art of War (Sun Tzu) 42, 43
assertiveness 77
assets 7, 8, 9, 128
assurance 16, 17
ASTM CCR (Continuity of Care Record) 55
Athens passwords 57
audit 2, 6, 29, 94
automated medical records 54
autonomy 67
avoidance 77
awareness campaigns 36

balance sheet 6, 8–9, 128
bank loans 7
bargaining 116
barriers to entry 45
Bass's model of transactional and transformational leadership 84
BCG (Boston Consulting Group) 47
Bebo 57
behaviour approach to leadership 82–3
Belbin Self-Perception Inventory 73
Belbin team roles 72–3, 80
benchmarking 62
Blackberry device 56
blogs 57, 58
Bolton Improving Care System 20, 27
bonuses 64
Boston Consulting Group (BCG) 47
Burns' model of transactional and transformational leadership 83
business process re-engineering 22–3
buyers 46

campaigns 36
cancer care 79
capital 45
carpal tunnel decompression surgery 23
case-based learning 108
Caseletto, JA 23

case studies
  accounting and finance 8
  clinical leaders 85
  human resource management 63, 67
  operations management 17, 18–19, 20,
    22, 23
  performance measurement 93–4
  strategic management 43, 50
cash flow 5, 6
cash flow statement 6, 10–11, 128
CCR (Continuity of Care Record) 55
CDA (Clinical Document Architecture) 55
CEN – EN13606 55
Centers for Disease Control and Prevention
    (CDC) 28, 41
champions 35, 36
Champy, J 22
change 115–22
  anatomy of management 2, 4
  change management 115–19
  definition 128
  exercises 122
  leading a successful change initiative
    119–21
  summary 121
  useful websites 122
  why change fails 119
charisma 84
Charted Institute of Marketing 41
Chartered Institute of Personnel and
    Development 90, 114
chief executives 124
CIRO framework (context, inputs, reactions,
    outcomes) 110
climate change 47
clinical audit 2, 94
Clinical Document Architecture (CDA) 55
Clinical Excellence Awards 124
clinical leaders 81–90
  becoming a transformational leader 85–6
  case studies 85
  clinical team 73, 78
  mentoring and coaching 86–9
  study of leadership 81–3
  transactional and transformational
    leadership 83–5
clinical performance 91
clinical team 69–80
  anatomy of a team 70
  building effective teams 73

conflict 75–8
definition 69, 128
delegation 74–5
exercises 79, 89
physiology of the clinical team 70–2
summary 79, 89
team dynamics 73–4
team effectiveness model 73
team roles 72–3
useful websites 80, 90
why the clinical team? 78–9
working examples 79
CMR (computerised medical record) 54
coaching 88–9, 128
collaborative delegation style 75
collaborators (five Cs of marketing) 29–30
Commonwealth Health Corporation,
    Kentucky 19
communication 76, 91, 119
Companies Act 6
company (five Cs of marketing) 29
company law 6
competitive advantage 48, 50
competitive rivalry 46–7
competitors (five Cs of marketing) 30
computerised medical record (CMR) 54
concentration 46
concrete experience 102, 103
conditioning 102
conflict 71, 73, 74, 75–8, 128
consumer demographic 31
consumer expectations 15, 16
context (five Cs of marketing) 30–1
contingency theory 83
contingent reward 85
Continuity of Care Record (CCR) 55
control 50
controlling delegation style 75
cooperativeness 77
copyrights 7, 45
corporations 6
cosmetic surgery 47
cost leadership strategy 47, 128
costs
  accounting and finance 9, 10
  operations management 15
  performance management 96
  strategic management 45
culture (definition) 128
current assets 7, 8, 128

customers 31, 35, 36
customer value 20

defect rates 18
delegation 73, 74–5, 128
demand-based assessment 62
demand-based pricing 34
Deming, W Edwards 20
denial of change 116
Department of Health 54, 97
dependability 14, 128
depreciation 7, 10
depression 116
DICOM standard 55
differentiation 45, 46, 48
direct costs 10
directors' report 6
discrimination 47
distribution channels 45
diversification 49, 50
dividends 10
DMAIC model (define, measure, analyse, improve, control) 18
doctors
    clinical team 79
    information technology 56
    innovation in medicine 124, 125–6
    performance management 91, 93, 94–5, 97–9
    why the clinical team? 78
dysfunctional conflict 75, 77, 78

economic climate 47
economies of scale 34, 45, 47
education 57, 119
effectiveness 128
efficiency ratios 11–12
e-learning 57, 102, 108–9
electronic health care record (EHCR) 54, 55
electronic health record (EHR) 55, 58
electronic medical record (EMR) 54, 55
electronic patient record (EPR) 54
empathy 16, 17
environment 47
equity 7, 8, 9, 11, 128
evaluation
    learning and teaching 110, 113
    operations management 22
    strategic management 50

exit barriers 46
expectations 15, 16, 17
expenses 2, 9, 10
experience curve 47
experiential learning model 102

Facebook 57, 58, 60
feedback 67, 73, 88, 95, 96, 110
final behavioural objectives 107
finance (definition) 5–6 see also accounting and finance
financial accounting 5 see also accounting and finance
financiers of healthcare 96–7
five Cs of marketing 29, 31
fixed assets 7, 8, 11, 128
fixed costs 9, 128
flexibility 15, 128
'flow' production 20
focus strategy 49
forming stage of team development 70
Fortune 1000 companies 119
forward integration 46
foundation trusts 6
4Ps of the marketing mix 32, 33
functional conflict 75, 77, 78

Galton, F 81
gap model 15–16
General Medical Council (GMC) 92, 96, 97, 101
good medical practice 92, 97–9, 123
goodwill 7
Google 55, 56, 57
government policy 45, 47
grants 29
grief stages 115
gross profit 10, 12

Hammer, M 22
handouts 107
Haslam, C 96
Healthcare Workforce Portal 68
health marketing 28–9
health promotion 3, 36
HealthVault 55
Heart Improvement Programme 27
Herzberg's motivation-hygiene theory 64–6
hip fractures 20
hiring 64

HISA standard 55
HL7 messages 55
holistic care 69
Honey and Mumford learner types 103, 104
hospitals 17
human resource management 61-8
  anatomy of management 2, 4
  case studies 63, 67
  exercises 68
  recruitment 63-4
  requirements of workforce 61-2
  retention of staff 64-7
  reward management 64
  strategic human resource management 61
  summary 67
  useful websites 68
  workforce planning 62
hygiene factors 65, 66

iCal 57
idealised influence 84
IFRS (International Financial Reporting
    Standards) 6
imaging 55-6
implementation of plans 50
income 2, 9, 10
incorporated companies 6
independent teams 70
indirect costs 10
individualised consideration 85
inflation 47
Information Technology Association of
    America (ITAA) 53
information technology (IT) 53-60
  anatomy of management 2, 3
  definition 53
  exercises 59
  imaging 55-6
  online education 57
  organisational level 59
  patient care 53-5
  performance management 97
  personal development 56
  research and information 56-7
  scheduling 57
  social networking 57-8
  summary 59
  useful websites 60
innovation in medicine 123-7
  anatomy of management 2, 4

definition 128
exercises 127
innovative doctor 125-6
innovative healthcare organisation
    124-5
innovative management 125
useful websites 127
inputs 13
inspirational motivation 84
intangible fixed assets 7, 128
integrative approach to leadership 83
interdependent teams 70
interim behavioural objectives 107
International Financial Reporting Standards
    (IFRS) 6
internet
  e-learning 57, 102, 108-9
  online education 57
  promotion 36
  research and information 56-7
  social networking 57-8
interviewing 64
intra-group conflict 71
Intute 56
investment 10
iPhone 56
Irvine, D 92
ISO 18308 55
ISO TC215 55
IT *see* information technology

Jacobs, K 97
job description 63, 125
job design 63
job enlargement 67, 128
job enrichment 67, 129
job rotation 67
job satisfaction 64-5, 67
Journal of the American Medical Association
    58
journals 56, 126

key performance indicators (KPIs) 93-4,
    125, 129
Kilmann, R 76, 77
knowledge, skill and ability (KSA) analysis
    106-7, 112
Kolb Learning Cycle 102, 103, 104
Kotler, P 29, 34, 39
Kotter, JP 120, 121

KSA (knowledge, skill and ability) analysis
106–7, 112
Kubler-Ross stages of grief 115, 117
Kumar, V 35

laissez-faire leadership 85
law 6
leadership *see* clinical leaders
Leading Change (Kotter) 120
Lean 20, 21, 119, 129
Lean Six Sigma 21–2, 129
learning and teaching 102–14
  exercises 111–14
  learning 102–3
  learning event planning 105–10
  summary 110
  types of learner 103–5
  useful websites 114
learning organisations 106
lectures 107
legislation 47
liabilities 7, 8, 9, 11, 129
licences 45, 96
limited liability companies 6
LinkedIn 57, 60
liquidity 7, 10
liquidity ratios 11
loans 7
Locke, EA 67
long-term liabilities 7
loss leader pricing 34

Maastricht University 108
management
  anatomy of 2–4
  applicability to clinical practice 1–2
  clinical team 78, 79
  definition 1, 129
  innovation in medicine 124, 125
  performance management 97
  study of leadership 83
management accounting 5
management by exception-active 85
management by exception-passive 85
managing clinicians' performance *see*
    performance management
market development 49, 50
marketing in healthcare 28–41
  analysis of marketing opportunities
    29–31

anatomy of management 2, 3
definition of marketing 28, 129
developing the marketing mix 32
exercises 37–40
managing the marketing effort 36–7
marketing and healthcare 28–9
marketing process 29
selecting target markets 31–2
summary 37
marketing mix 32, 129
market penetration 49, 50
market segmentation 31–2, 129
market targeting 32
Maslow's hierarchy of needs 64, 66,
  129
McCarthy, EJ 32
McKneally, MF 123
media advertising 36
medical education 58, 123
medical records 54, 55, 58
Medical Records Institute 54
medical research 123
medical schools 58, 123
MEDLINE® 56
melanoma 93–4
mentoring 86–8, 129
MeSH (Medical Subject Headings) 56
Michigan University 82, 83
Microsoft 55, 57
microsurgery 112–14
minimum wage 47
misconduct 91
misers 35, 36
monopoly 46
mortality rates 20
motion capture analysis 22
motivation 84
motivation-hygiene theory 64–6
Motorola 18
Moullin, Max 91
multi-source feedback (MSF) 95
Mumford, A 103, 104

National Library of Medicine 56
needs assessment 62, 105–7, 112
net cash flow 10
net profit 10
NHS (National Health Service)
  accounting and finance 6
  information technology 53, 57

NHS (National Health Service) – (*contd*)
  innovation in medicine 124
  operations management 17
  workforce planning 62
NHS Connecting for Health 60, 114, 122
NHS Information Centre 68
NHS Institute for Innovation and
    Improvement 21, 27, 90, 101, 127
NHS Leadership Qualities Framework 90
niche market 49
Nine Price/Quality Pricing Strategies 34,
    35, 39
norming stage of team development 71
nurses 78, 125

objective setting 14–16, 42–3, 107
Ohio State University 82
oligopoly 46
online education 57, 102, 108–9
open EHR (electronic health record) 55
operating profit 10
operation costs 15
operations management 13–26
  anatomy of management 2–3
  case studies 17, 18–19, 20, 22, 23, 26
  definition 129
  employment of methods to improve
      performance 18–23
    Lean 20
    Lean Six Sigma 21–2
    process re-engineering 22–3
    Six Sigma 18–19
  exercises 24–6
  managing activities required to create and
      deliver goods or services 13–14
  substantial measurement and analysis of
      processes 14–17
  summary 24
  useful websites 27
opportunity costs 9, 129
organisational analysis 106, 112
organisational culture 62, 117–18, 129
orthopaedic care 37–9
Outlook 57
outpatient team 79
outputs 13, 14

PACS *see* Picture Archiving and
    Communications System
parallel pricing 46

Parasuraman consumer expectation-
    perception gap model 15–16
participative delegation style 75
participative leadership 83
patents 7, 45
pathology 18
Patient Administration System (PAS) 53
patient care 53–5
patient pathway 79, 91, 92–3
patients
  innovation in medicine 125
  performance management 95–6
  satisfaction 16, 17, 95, 96
Pavlov's dogs 102
pay 64
PBL *see* problem-based learning
PCPI *see* Physician Consortium for
    Performance Improvement
peer review 94
perceptions 15, 16, 17
performance management 91–101
  anatomy of management 2, 3
  case studies 93–4
  definition of performance 91, 129
  exercises 100
  human resource management 64
  key performance indicators 93–4
  managing doctors' performance 97–9
  patient pathway 92–3
  summary 99
  useful websites 101
  what is measured 91–2
  what matters most 94
  who drives performance? 94–7
  why manage performance? 94
  workforce planning 62
performance objectives 14–16
performing stage of team development 71
personal development 56
personal health records 58
personal information managers (PIMs) 57
personalisation 76
person analysis 107
PESTEL (Political, Economic, Social,
    Technological, Environmental, Legal)
    analysis 30, 47, 48, 129
Peters, TJ 124
pharmaceuticals 126
Physician Consortium for Performance
    Improvement (PCPI) 92, 93

Picker Institute 95
Picture Archiving and Communications
    System (PACS) 18–19, 55
PIMS (personal information managers) 57
place 34
plans 47–50
plastic surgery 85
podcasts 57
point of sale 35
political factors 47
population-based estimating 62
Porter's five forces 36, 43–7, 129
Porter's strategies 47–9, 129
power-influence approach to leadership 83
power of buyers 46
power of suppliers 45–6
Prabhu, Jaideep 126
pragmatist learning style 104
Price/Quality Pricing Strategies 34, 35, 39
price sensitivity 46
primary care trusts 94
private sector 28
problem-based learning (PBL) 108, 109
process conflict 75
processes in change 118–19
process mapping 22, 23, 25
process re-engineering 22–3, 119, 129
product 32–4
product development 49, 50
product differentiation 45, 46, 48
product life cycle 32–4, 129
professional development 57
professionalism 92
profitability ratios 12
profit and loss account 6, 9–10, 129
profit formula 9
promotion 35–6
psychographics 32
public relations 35
public sector 28–9, 36
PubMed 56

quality 2, 15–16, 129
Quality and Outcomes Framework 96
quality improvement methodologies 18–23
quality indicators 94
questionnaires 95, 96

radiology 18, 19, 55
Rajaratnam, V 23

ranking 64
ratio analysis 2, 11–12
recruitment 63–4, 65
re-design 25
referencing 64
reflective observation 102, 103
reflector learning style 104
regulatory bodies 96
relationship conflict 75
relations-orientated behaviour 83
reliability 16, 17
requirements analysis 106
requirements of workforce 61–2
research 29, 56–7, 123, 126
ResearchGate 126, 127
resistance to change 116–20
resources 2, 13, 62
responsiveness 16, 17
resuscitation 72
retention of staff 64–7
revalidation 96
revenue 9
reward management 64
road accidents 39
Rodger, JA 97
Rosenberg, N 123
Royal Bolton Hospital NHS Foundation
    Trust 27

salaries 64
sales 9
scans 55
scheduling 57
SCU *see* strategic clinical unit
search engines 56
Senge, PM 106
service quality models 15–16, 17
SERVQUAL scale 16, 17, 92, 93
'seven jump step' model 108, 109
sexual misconduct 91
short-listing 64
short-term liabilities 7
SHRM *see* strategic human resource
    management
simulation-based learning 108
situational approach to leadership 83
Six Sigma 18–19, 21, 119, 130
skill 106
skimming 34
small group teaching 107–8

SMART objectives 42, 130
smart phones 56
social networking 57–8
social trends 47
software 55
solvency 10
solvency ratios 11
speed 14, 130
staffing requirements 61–2
staff retention 64–7
stages of change 115–16
statement of total recognised gains and
    losses 6
stock turnover 11
Stodgill, RM 81
storming stage of team development 71
strategic clinical unit (SCU) 69, 79, 125,
    130
strategic human resource management
    (SHRM) 61, 130
strategic management 42–53
    analysis 43
    case studies 43, 50
    evaluation and control 50
    exercises 51
    implementation of plan 50
    objective setting 42–3
    PESTEL 47
    plans 47–50
    Porter's five forces 43–7
    strategic process 51
    strategy 42
    summary 50
    SWOT analysis 43, 44
strategy 2, 3, 42, 130
substantial measurement and analysis of
    processes 14–17
substitutes 45
sunk costs 9, 130
Sun Tzu 42, 43
suppliers 45–6
surgical process re-engineering 22, 23, 70
SWOT (Strengths, Weaknesses,
    Opportunities, Threats) analysis 30,
    43, 44, 130

tangible fixed assets 7, 128
tangibles 16, 17
target audience 107
target markets 31–2

task conflict 75
task-orientated behaviour 83
task significance 67
taxation 10, 47
Taylor, FW 20
team approach 86, 123, 125 *see also* clinical
    team
team effectiveness model 73, 74
team roles 72–3
technology 47
tentative delegation style 75
theorist learning style 104
Thibodaux Regional Medical Center 19
Thomas and Kilmann conflict responses
    76, 77
threat of entry 45
threat of substitutes 45
360-degree feedback 95
time management 56, 57
tips 64
Toyota 20
training-output estimating 62
trait approach to leadership 81–2
transactional leadership 83, 84, 85
transformational leadership 83, 84–6
transformation process 13, 14
transformed resources 13, 14
transforming resources 13, 14
trauma care 22, 37–40
Tuckman's stages of team development
    70–1
turnover 9, 62, 64, 130
Twitter 57, 58, 60
two-factor theory (Herzberg) 64–6

University of Maastricht 108
University of Michigan 82, 83
University of Victoria team effectiveness
    model 73, 74
university websites 56

value stream 20
variable costs 9, 130
Victoria University team effectiveness model
    73, 74
videos 57
virtual learning environments (VLEs) 57,
    109
vision 86

Warr, P 110
waste 20
Waterman, RH 124
weather 47
word of mouth 15, 35
workforce planning 62, 130
working capital 11

X-rays 55

Youssef, F 17

Zavod, MB 35
Zlotnik-Shaul, R 123